Simulators in
Anesthesiology Education

Simulators in Anesthesiology Education

Edited by

Lindsey C. Henson and
Andrew C. Lee

University of Rochester School of Medicine and Dentistry
Rochester, New York

Plenum Press • New York and London

Library of Congress Cataloging-in-Publication Data

Simulators in anesthesiology education / edited by Lindsey C. Henson
and Andrew C. Lee.
          p.   cm.
     "Proceedings of the Second Annual Conference on Simulators in
Anesthesiology Education, held May 31-June 2, 1996, in Rochester,
New York"--T.p. verso.
     Includes bibliographical references and index.
     ISBN 0-306-45775-X
     1. Anesthesiology--Study and teaching--Simulation methods-
-Congresses. 2. Athesthesia--Computer simulation--Congresses.
I. Henson, Lindsey C. II. Lee, Andrew C. III. Conference on
Simulators in Anesthesiology Education (2nd : 1996 : Rochester,
N.Y.)
     [DNLM: 1. Anesthesiology--education--congresses. 2. Computer
Simulation--congresses. 3. Teaching--methods--congresses.   WO 218
S614 1997]
RD80.7.S57 1997
617.9'6'0785--dc21
DNLM/DLC
for Library of Congress   97-46469
                                                                 CIP

Proceedings of the Second Annual Conference on Simulators in Anesthesiology Education, held May 31–June 2, 1996, in Rochester, New York

ISBN 0-306-45775-X

© 1998 Plenum Press, New York
A Division of Plenum Publishing Corporation
233 Spring Street, New York, N.Y. 10013

http://www.plenum.com

10 9 8 7 6 5 4 3 2 1

Printed in the United States of America

PREFACE

In the past ten years, full-scale simulation training has become dramatically more evident in undergraduate and graduate medical education. This increase has been due primarily to two factors: the development of new computer-driven technology and an interest in simulation-specific training techniques. Technologically, simulators have evolved from simple anatomical reproductions to full-scale accurate reproductions of anatomy and physiology powered by multiple computers. High-technology simulation centers run by teams of faculty are emerging as integral tools in fulfilling medical centers' educational missions. In addition, educational techniques specific to simulation, which have been developed and used by other industries for over half a century, are being applied to medical training.

Aviation and aerospace have used sophisticated simulation since the 1950s to train pilots and astronauts. Extrapolating these methods for use in the medical world has been a natural course of events, particularly in specialties that require some of the same basic thought processes and interactions required of the pilot or astronaut. It is not surprising, then, that anesthesiology would be the medical specialty to take the lead in adding simulation training to its educational programs. The anesthesiologist's job in the operating room is similar to that of a pilot in a cockpit, not in the specific tasks, but in decision making, technological and human interfaces, and crisis management.

Modern simulation of the anesthesiologist's working environment is getting closer and closer to reality. The appearance and sounds of the patient, the monitor readouts, and the entire operating room environment can be re-created in a full-scale simulation center. This high-fidelity simulated environment allows the opportunity for a variety of training exercises. These range from the simple study of physiologic principles and practice of specific procedures to more complex decision-making exercises and crisis management. Rare problems or events that an anesthesiologist might never experience during a residency training program can be repeatedly practiced and analyzed in the simulation center.

The real value in simulation, however, lies in the ability to help members of the operating room team develop systematic approaches to decision making and action. If these approaches to problems can be developed in the controlled simulated environment, without putting real patients at risk, it is hoped that they will be applied to real cases and possibly effect real changes in outcome.

In this era of cost containment, cutbacks, and litigation, one may question whether this high-technology, expensive training is worthwhile. The end result of simulation training may be medical practice of higher "quality" and "safety" that, in the end, saves both time and money. Moreover, the increasing load of material that medical students or residents must learn has become overwhelming, especially with their duties in clinical patient care. Simulation education may actually help condense material through specific programs that allow participants to experience challenging situations on a more concentrated level. Finally, new areas of education such as team training and crisis management can be offered exclusively in the simulated environment. It is still too early to be able to answer the question of whether simulation training is "worth it" but the answer is vital to the continued growth of the field.

The purpose of this book is to present work that has been done over the past several years in the area of simulation in anesthesiology education. The chapters come from presentations given at the Second Annual Conference on Simulators in Anesthesiology Education in Rochester, New York. The conference took place from May 31–June 2, 1996 and the participants represented an international community of physicians, nurses, technicians, and educators interested in this new field. Presentations and workshops covered a wide range of topics from specific hardware concerns, programming techniques, and educational applications, to research in naturalistic environments and crisis resource management. Dr. Robert Helmreich provided the keynote address regarding human factors in medicine.

We would like to thank Dr. Alice Basford for her determination, enthusiasm, and organizational efforts, which made the Conference so successful. We also express our appreciation to the organizations that provided contributions to the Conference (CAE Electronics, Inc., Medical Education Technologies, Inc., and Glaxo-Wellcome), to Ms. Pamela Dougherty for her excellent administrative efforts in planning the conference and preparation of this volume, and to the other staff in the Department of Anesthesiology at the University of Rochester who helped with the conference.

Hopefully, this book will provide a point of reference for where the science of simulation currently is, and an inspiration for those who see the great potential for the future of this new modality.

A. C. Lee
L. C. Henson

CONTENTS

1. Turning Silk Purses into Sows' Ears: Human Factors in Medicine   1
   Robert L. Helmreich and Hans-Gerhard Schäfer

2. Teaching High School Students   9
   W. Bosseau Murray and Arthur J. L. Schneider

3. Integration of the Human Patient Simulator into the Medical Student
      Curriculum: Life Support Skills 15
   Eugene B. Freid

4. Using Simulators for Medical Students and Anesthesia Resident Education 23
   Andrew C. Lee

5. Simulation in Nursing Anesthesia Education: Practical and Conceptual
      Perspectives 29
   Alfred E. Lupien

6. What Can You Do with a Simulator?: Quality Assurance 39
   Vimal Chopra

7. Team Orientated Medical Simulation 51
   Stephan C. U. Marsch

8. Workshop on Educational Aspects: Educational Objectives and Building
      Scenarios 57
   W. Bosseau Murray and Lindsey C. Henson

9. Model Driven Simulators from the Clinical Instructor's Perspective: Current
      Status and Evolving Concepts 65
   Willem L. van Meurs and Tammy Y. Euliano

10. Technical Workshop: Mathematical and Computer Models 75
    David H. Stern

11. Issues in Starting a Simulator Program 85
    Barry L. Zimmerman

12. Research Techniques in Human Performance Using Realistic Simulation 93
    David M. Gaba

13. Performance Enhancement in Anesthesia Using the Training Simulator Sophus
    (Peanuts) 103
    John Jacobsen, Per F. Jensen, Doris Ostergaard, Astrid Lindekær,
    Anne Lippert, and Peter Schultz

14. Jumpseating in the Operating Room 107
    B. Sexton, S. Marsch, R. Helmreich, D. Betzendoerfer, T. Kocher,
    D. Scheidegger, and the TOMS team

15. Participant Evaluation of Team Oriented Medical Simulation 109
    B. Sexton, S. Marsch, R. Helmreich, D. Betzendoerfer, T. Kocher,
    D. Scheidegger, and the TOMS team

16. Evaluation of Simulator Use for Anesthesia Resident Orientation 111
    D. M. Barron and R. K. Russell

17. Incorporation of a Realistic Anesthesia Simulator into an Anesthesia Clerkship .. 115
    M. Pamela Fish and Brendan Flanagan

18. Computer Analysis of Cerebrovascular Hemodynamics during Induction of
    Anesthesia 121
    A. Bekker, S. Wolk, H. Turndorf, and A. Ritter

Index 123

TURNING SILK PURSES INTO SOWS' EARS

Human Factors in Medicine

Robert L. Helmreich and Hans-Gerhard Schäfer

[1]Department of Psychology
University of Texas at Austin
[2]Department of Anesthesia
University of Basel/Kantonsspital

This paper describes lessons learned from research into team behavior and the interpersonal roots of accidents and incidents in aviation. This research has led to the development of training programs, known as Crew Resource Management, that are mandated for flight crews worldwide. Approaches to developing similar programs for medical personnel working in operating and emergency rooms are described.

1. SUPERMAN IN THE COCKPIT AND THE OPERATING ROOM

Many physicians, like pilots, maintain unrealistic views of their personal capabilities under stressful conditions. Members of both professions tend to deny that their performance and decision making are adversely affected by fatigue, pressure, or working with less capable associates. They also vigorously endorse the statement that 'A true professional can leave personal problems behind when (entering the cockpit) entering the OR.' It can perhaps be argued that such a sense of invulnerability may be useful on the battlefield where generals would like their fighter pilots to attack relentlessly without regard for personal danger and to be concerned with victory not survival. In the case of medicine and commercial aviation, however, there would seem to be few benefits and many risks associated with feeling oneself impervious to mortal challenges. Research data provide strong evidence to the contrary: individuals under high stress are more likely to make decision errors, to be less capable of processing multiple inputs, and less likely to maintain high levels of vigilance and situation awareness. Fortunately, these attitudes can be modified by training that includes the scientific evidence regarding the limitations of human performance. Figure 1 shows the percentage of pilots from a major U.S. airline and combined OR staff from three countries who agree with the statement 'Even when fatigued, I perform effectively during critical phases (of flight) of operations.' The 1988 data for pilots show attitudes before any training on the effects of stressors. The far right column shows the

Simulators in Anesthesiology Education, edited by Henson and Lee.
Plenum Press, New York, 1998.

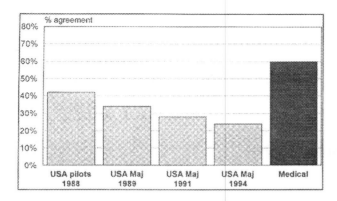

Figure 1. Percent agreement with the statement "Even when fatigued, I perform effectively during (critical times of flight) critical phases of operations" in aviation and medicine.

attitudes of surgeons, anesthesiologists and nurses without training. It is noteworthy that the baseline medical attitudes are even more unrealistic than those of pilots.

One of the goals of human factors training is to give individuals a more realistic appraisal of their capabilities—hence the obscure message in the title. In aviation, it is to turn Sky Gods into Mortals—silk purses, if you will, into sows' ears. The good news, shown in Figure 1 with data from 1989 through 1994, is that attitudes shift over time with exposure to training and individuals come to accept their limitations and to recognize the value of teams and communications as countermeasures against the error.[1]

2. LESSONS FROM AVIATION

NASA research into the causes of crashes in commercial aviation revealed that human error is a causal factor in the majority of accidents and critical incidents.[2] Further investigation demonstrated that the majority of human error involved failures in leadership, communication, decision making and vigilance rather than technical errors in the operation of systems or equipment. Examination of training practices further indicated that pilots' actions reflected their training in the execution of individual technical skills with little emphasis on the teamwork involved in managing a complex aircraft with a multi-person crew. These data suggested that the emphasis in training may have been misplaced and the industry responded by initiating a new approach to qualifying pilots.

2.1. The Development of CRM

Training in teamwork and communications skills (sometimes called interpersonal human factors) was developed by several U.S. airlines during the early 1980s. These programs were known initially as Cockpit Resource Management (CRM). They normally have two major components, interactive seminars where relevant human factors concepts are presented and discussed (for example, limitations on human performance under stressful conditions; group decision strategies, etc.) and simulator training where crews fly a complete mission under highly realistic conditions. This type of training, known as Line Oriented Flight Training (LOFT), represents a departure from the original use of flight simulators to train individuals in technical maneuvers toward their employment to train and reinforce interpersonal, team skills. One of the central features of LOFT is the use of video recordings to capture interactions for later debriefing and instruction in the dynamics of flight management.[2]

During the last fifteen years, CRM training has evolved steadily into a highly focused approach to instruction and reinforcement that deals both with specific behaviors related to successful team performance and also with understanding of system and organizational factors that form the environment in which crews function. One of the major changes has been to broaden the scope of the team from the cockpit to include those with whom pilots must interact in managing flight—cabin personnel, ground support, and air traffic control. Reflecting this change in scope, the name has changed from *Cockpit* to *Crew Resource Management*, although the algorithm has remained constant. The Crew model is closer to the situation of the Operating Room (OR) which is staffed by teams from different disciplines.[2]

Our research group at the University of Texas at Austin has been involved in the development and evaluation of CRM programs since their inception. One of our major tasks has been to determine the operational impact of these programs and their limitations.[3] The data allow a number of conclusions to be drawn about utility of human factors training. First, it should be noted that in aviation, as in medicine, the frequency of catastrophic events is low. Because the number of accidents is (happily) so low, it would take many years to draw inferences about the impact of a program on the accident rate. As a result, multiple, surrogate criterion measures are employed. These include measures of participant attitudes and reactions to training, expert observations of behavior in operational settings, and data on incidents (positive and negative). From data accumulated in more than 30 organizations in sixteen countries, we can conclude that CRM training is enthusiastically received by participants and is effective in changing attitudes and behavior. Based on accumulating evidence demonstrating effectiveness, CRM is being required for commercial airline pilots throughout the world. The evidence, however, is not uniformly positive. A number of factors have been isolated that limit the impact of programs. One of the most critical is organizational commitment. If the organizational culture is not supportive of team concepts and open communication, training will not change operational behavior. Second, programs need to be data driven. That is, they need to be based on data that indicate the strengths and weaknesses of the particular organization rather than being generic, off the shelf training packages. Third, leaders in the organization need special training in human factors and the evaluation of performance so they can become role models and agents to reinforce desired behaviors. Fourth, programs must be ongoing and not one-shot interventions. Continuing assessment is required to determine areas of strength and areas in need of further attention. Fifth, programs need to address human factors at multiple levels: at the system level by showing how behavior and performance are constrained by organizational and environmental factors, at the group level by providing instruction in effective communication, leadership, and team coordination, and at the individual level by providing instruction in individual limits on performance (for example, the impact of stressors, as discussed earlier).

3. RELATING CRM TO MEDICINE

A number of anesthesiologists saw parallels between crew training and simulation in aviation and the practice of anesthesia. They recognized that failures in communication could have common roots in both the cockpit and the OR. The potential of simulators for training was also noted and anesthesia simulator facilities with associated training programs have been constructed in Europe and Asia as well as the United States.[4,5,6,7,8]

3.1. The Multiple Functions of Simulators

Both in aviation and in medicine, simulators can be used to serve different purposes and the distinctions among these uses are important to note. Table 1 shows the three primary uses of simulators in both domains.

The first use made of simulators in aviation was to train individual pilots in technical maneuvers such as landings and steep turns. In medicine, an anesthesia simulator can be used to give residents and students practice in intubation and use of anesthesia machines. One of the advantages of simulation in both domains is that neither patients nor passengers are placed at risk; the consequences of error are minimal. This form of simulation is frequently described as *part-task simulation* since only part of an array of tasks is being practiced. A more comprehensive approach to simulation has become known as *SPOT* or *Special Purpose Operational Training*. In aviation, this type of simulation includes a complete crew (pilot, co-pilot and, if a non-automated aircraft, a flight engineer) who practice critical maneuvers where team coordination is required. In anesthesia, this type of simulation was developed by David Gaba and his colleagues and has become known as Anesthesia Crisis Resource Management (ACRM) training.[9] ACRM is conducted in a simulated operating room with an instrumented mannequin. The anesthesia staff (attendings, residents, etc.) conduct the anesthesia under realistic conditions with one major exception: the roles of the surgical staff are played by actors as there is no capability in the simulation facility for surgical procedures to be conducted. The most advanced simulation in aviation has come to be known as *LOFT* or *Line Oriented Flight Training*.[10] *LOFT* represents the highest level of fidelity in simulation, with all aspects of flight being presented from paperwork to air traffic control and all crewmembers having meaningful tasks to complete. This type of simulation in medicine, involving all OR personnel from surgeons to orderlies, has become known as *Team Oriented Medical Simulation* or *TOMS*. The remainder of this discussion will focus on integrated human factors training and *TOMS* as a means of enhancing teamwork in the OR.

4. DEVELOPING AN INTEGRATED HUMAN FACTORS PROGRAM

The late Hans-Gerhard Schäfer of the Department of Anaesthesia, University of Basel/Kantonsspital was one of the earliest to recognize the potential of human factors programs in anesthesia. Schäfer began by immersing himself in the aviation operational and research setting. As a Visiting Scientist at the University of Texas at Austin, he became familiar with the major programs in U.S. commercial aviation and also with the research tools and methodologies being used to investigate crew performance and measure

Table 1. Three levels of simulation in medicine and aviation

Aviation	Medicine
Part-task simulation	Part-task simulation
• Procedures	• Procedures
Special Purpose Operational Training (SPOT)	Anesthesia Crisis Resource Management (ACRM)
• Critical events	• Critical events
• Partial team	• Partial team
Line Oriented Flight Training (LOFT)	Team Oriented Medical Simulation (TOMS)
• Whole flight simulation	• Whole OR simulation

the impact of training. Following this exposure, the first author was invited to Basel for similar exposure to the human factors of the OR.

Our initial approach the dynamics of the OR was to observe operations in progress to determine if there were problems in communication and shared awareness. Noting that the difficulties observed were highly similar to those found in the cockpit, we proceeded to design a survey instrument to assess acceptance of human factors concepts and recognition of personal limitations. These data convinced us that OR teams would benefit significantly from exposure to training conceptually similar to CRM.[11]

There was support from the departments of anaesthesia and surgery for the development of joint human factors training and Schäfer headed a team of volunteers to turn the desire into reality. A four phase program, of which simulation was a part, was developed that paralleled the most modern CRM approaches in aviation.

4.1. Phase 1: Diagnosis

The first phase of the program consisted of diagnosis of the organization, not only to verify that training was needed, but also to determine what topics should be stressed in the curriculum. This was accomplished through a survey, the Operating Room Management Attitudes Questionnaire (ORMAQ) that was adapted from a questionnaire widely used in aviation.[12] The survey was completed by more than two-thirds of the staff (nurses, anesthesiologists, surgeons) of the departments of anesthesia and surgery. Results indicated that there were significant differences among the groups in attitudes regarding communication and leadership. The data also showed a reluctance on the part of many to question the actions and decisions of superiors. Responses to an open ended question about the major need to improve the safety and efficiency of the OR overwhelmingly identified better communication as the central concern. Figure 2 provides anecdotal evidence that, at least in the U.S., relations between surgery and anesthesia are sometimes sub-optimal.

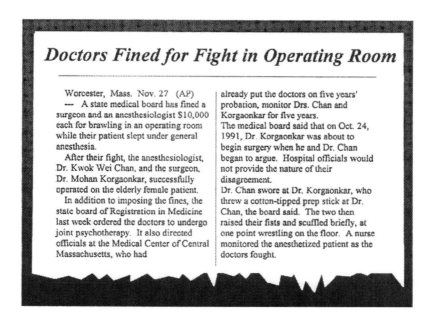

Figure 2. Conflict resolution in the operating room.

Observations had also identified interface issues among the OR's groups (for example, between surgeons and anesthesiologists) as a major source of conflict and misunderstanding. The data provided sufficient confirmation to embark on the second phase of the program.

4.2. Phase 2: Curriculum Design and Development

A first task was to develop materials for seminar discussion that demonstrate the importance of human factors and the ubiquity of human error. This presentation also included specifically defined behaviors that can enhance or impede effective communication and team coordination. Major topics include briefings and debriefings, decision processes, situation awareness, and the effects of stress and fatigue. Further instruction was developed for a one day seminar for departmental senior leadership. An additional program was developed for attendings to include focus on issues of performance evaluation and resident training.

The heart of the program was a full OR simulator that combined an anesthetic mannequin with a laparoscopic simulator to allow both surgical and anesthesia teams to perform meaningful work requiring inter-team coordination. The anesthetic mannequin, named of course, Wilhelm Tell, to reflect his Helvetic origins, was controlled by a PC based system developed by the Sophus group in Copenhagen, Denmark. The system contained models for various drugs as well as reactions such as tachycardia for the patient. The simulator facility also includes a control room with one way glass into the 'operating' room. The simulation is managed from the control room, which includes the computer control for the anesthesia simulator and video recording equipment to tape interactions in the OR as well as the laparoscopic procedure.[13]

TOMS training in the simulator is scheduled as though the simulator was a normal OR and assignment to TOMS is similar to assignment for a regular operation. The simulation includes a review of the patient's record and X-rays as well as discussion of the human factors concepts included in the simulation.

After the simulation is completed, the team assembles in an adjacent conference room and a guided discussion of the operation is conducted. This includes review of the videotapes of the operation to define and discuss critical group processes during the simulation.

4.3. Phase 3: Evaluation and Validation

One of the central research tasks is to determine the impact of training. To accomplish this, multiple criterion measures are collected. One of the essential criteria is the reaction of participants to the training itself. It can be argued that if participants reject the training, it is unlikely to have the desired effect. Reactions to training in Basel have been highly positive.[14] An ongoing quality assurance program also provides data on patient reactions and problems. A third source of information comes from systematic observation of team behavior in the OR through the use of expert observers trained to evaluate the behaviors addressed in training.[15] A fourth type of data comes from a newly developed Critical Incident Reporting System (CIRS) that allows personnel to input anonymous incident reports on an Intranet in the hospital.[16] Finally, by repeating the survey initially administered to obtain pre-training data, shifts in attitude can be assessed. These multiple data sources provide not only a report card on the program but also specific guidance for the focus of recurring training.

4.4. Phase 4: Continuing Training and Reinforcement

The fourth phase reflects the ongoing nature of human factors efforts. Training in both seminar and simulator continues. Particular emphasis is placed on evaluating and reinforcing the interpersonal aspects of medicine, both in the simulator and in the OR. Special focus continues to be addressed to the inter-team aspects of behavior.

5. SUMMARY AND CONCLUSIONS

The program at Basel is still in its infancy and data to validate its impact are still being collected. It can be concluded that the reactions of participants clearly support the utility of the effort. Simulation alone is not likely to produce major changes in attitudes and behavior, but embedded programs that address the array of interpersonal issues in medicine should have a higher probability of success.[17] The fact that the interpersonal difficulties in the OR strongly parallel those observed in the cockpit gives additional reason to believe that a program adapted from aviation but focused on observed issues in the OR will be as successful as those in aviation.

ACKNOWLEDGMENTS

The ability of the late Hans-Gerhard Schäfer of the Department of Anesthesia, The University of Basel/Kantonsspital to see the connections in seemingly diverse areas of science and his insights into the complexities of organizational and professional cultures have made an extraordinary contribution to medicine and psychology. I am also grateful to Dr. Daniel Scheidegger, Chairman of the Department of Anaesthesia and Dr. Felix Harder, Chairman of the Department of Surgery, both of whom have provided support and encouragement for the development of human factors in the hospital. Following Dr. Schäfer's death, the team of volunteers working with the human factors program gave unstintingly of their time and energy that the project would continue. I would like to thank the following members of the *TOMS* team: Dieter Betzendoerfer, Christoph Harms, Stephan Marsch, Olaf Schellscheidt, Christoph Schori, and Klaus Von Bulow. Particular thanks are due my students, Bryan Sexton and William Hines of the Department of Psychology of the University of Texas at Austin for their efforts in the program and to Dr. Jan M. Davies of the University of Calgary, Foothills Hospital for her constant encouragement and cogent critiques. The research of Robert Helmreich in aviation that provided background for the project was supported by NASA and by the Federal Aviation Administration.

REFERENCES

1. Helmreich, RL, Merritt, AC, Sherman, PJ: Human factors and national culture. ICAO J in press
2. Helmreich RL, Foushee HC. Why crew resource management? Empirical and theoretical bases of human factors training in aviation. *Cockpit Resource Management.* Edited by Wiener E, Kanki B, Helmreich RL. San Diego, Academic 1993; pp 3–45
3. Helmreich RL, Wilhelm JA. Outcomes of crew resource management training. *Int J Aviat Psych.* 1991; 1:287–300
4. Good ML, Lampotang S, Gibby GL, Gravenstein JS. Critical events simulation for training in anesthesiology. *J Clin Monit* 1988; 4:140

5. Gaba DM, DeAnda A. A comprehensive anesthesia simulating environment re-creating the operating room for research and training. *Anesthesiology* 1988; 69:387–94
6. Good ML, Gravenstein JS, Mahla ME, White SE, Banner MJ, Carovano RG, Lampotang S. Anaesthesia simulator for learning basic skills. *J Clin Monit* 1992; 8:187–8
7. Asbury AJ. Simulators for general anaesthesia. *Br J Anaesth* 1994; 73:285–286
8. Chopra V, Engbers FHM, Geerts MJ, Filet WR, Bovill JG, Spierdijk J. The Leiden anaesthesia simulator. *Br J Anaesth* 1994; 73:287–92
9. Howard SK, Gaba DM, Fish KJ, Yang G, Sarnquist FH. Anesthesia crisis resource management training: teaching anesthesiologists to handle critical incidents. *Aviat Space Environ Med* 1992; 63:763–70
10. Butler RE. LOFT: Full-mission simulation as crew resource management. *Cockpit Resource Management.* Edited by Wiener E, Kanki B, Helmreich RL. San Diego, Academic 1993, pp 199–223
11. Helmreich RL, Schäfer HG. Team performance in the operating room. In: Bogner MS (Ed.) *Human Error in Medicine,* Hillsdale, New Jersey, Erlbaum 1994; pp225–253
12. Helmreich RL, Merritt AC, Sherman PJ, Gregorich SE, & Wiener EL. The Flight Management Attitudes Questionnaire (FMAQ). 1993:NASA/UT/FAA Technical Report 93–1
13. Helmreich RL, & Davies JM. Human factors in the operating room: Interpersonal determinants of safety, efficiency and morale. In A.A. Aitkenhead (Ed.), *Bailliere's Clinical Anaesthesiology: Safety and Risk Management in Anaesthesia.* London: Balliere Tindall; 1996; pp277–296
14. Sexton, B., Marsch, S., Helmreich, R.L., Betzendoerfer, D., Kocher, T. & Scheidegger, D. (in press). Participant evaluations of Team Oriented Medical Simulation. In L. Henson, A. Lee, & A. Basford (Eds.) *Simulators in Anesthesiology Education.* New York. Plenum
15. Sexton, B., Marsch, S., Helmreich, R.L., Betzendoerfer, D., Kocher, T. & Scheidegger, D. (in press). Jumpseating in the Operating Room. In L. Henson, A. Lee, & A. Basford (Eds.) *Simulators in Anesthesiology Education.* New York. Plenum
16. Staender, S. Critical Incident Reporting System (CIRS), 1996; http://www.medana.unibas.ch/ENG/CIRS/Cirs.htm
17. Davies JM, Helmreich RL. Simulation: it's a start. *Can J Anaesth.* 1996;43:425–9

2

TEACHING HIGH SCHOOL STUDENTS

W. Bosseau Murray and Arthur J. L. Schneider

The Simulation Development and Cognitive Science Laboratory
Pennsylvania State University
College of Medicine
Milton S. Hershey Medical Center

1. INTRODUCTION

Computer controlled electro-mechanical human simulators are fascinating devices for which investigators have sought wide application. Here, we describe the use of a full human simulator to enrich the science lab experiences of high school students. Our intent is to describe the background and facilities of the "Education Lab" at the Pennsylvania State University College of Medicine and to describe in some detail how simulator scenarios were developed for high school students. The students who attended these scenario demonstrations were asked to complete an evaluative questionnaire at the end of the sessions. Their responses gave us insight into their needs, interests, and enthusiasm and are also reported here.

2. BACKGROUND

The Simulation Development and Cognitive Science Laboratory (Education Lab) was inaugurated in 1993 based on ideas and perceived needs expressed by the faculty of the Department of Anesthesiology. In July 1995, a full human simulator (Loral-Gainesville) was acquired through a cooperative effort of the Departments of Anesthesia, Nursing and Surgery. These three departments have remained the main users of the simulation mannequin and laboratory. Education lab experiences are also part of the educational activities of the Departments of Emergency Medicine and Internal Medicine. At the time of this report, the laboratory has a full time simulator technician, a full time automation engineer/computer specialist and instructional input from the clinical faculty of the involved departments.

Within the Department of Anesthesiology, a Director of the Laboratory heads an Education Laboratory Committee which works closely with the Computer and Library Committees. An Interdepartmental Committee coordinates activities of the three supporting departments, such as schedules, budgets, educational goals, and projects to be undertaken.

Simulators in Anesthesiology Education, edited by Henson and Lee.
Plenum Press, New York, 1998.

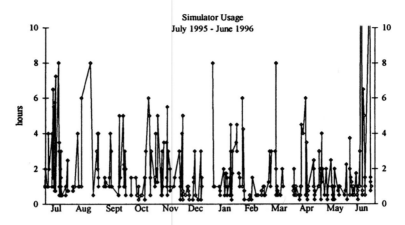

Figure 1. Simulator usage June 1995–June 1996.

3. UTILIZATION

Since both the capital investment and the salary cost of maintenance personnel for a full human simulator are considerable, there was interest in carefully monitoring the actual daily usage of the device. The mannequin averaged 2.5 hours per day of use over the first nine month period (see Figure 1). This listing does not include use of the other facilities in the lab, such as intubation and central venous access mannequins, educational computer programs and an interactive computer workstation, during those months. Use tended to be episodic as one group or another developed and utilized an educational experience for a particular group of students (Murray 1994).

The education laboratory concept was well received from the beginning. A few months after the lab was founded it won the Anesthesia Patient Safety Foundation award for a scientific display best demonstrating safety education at the 1993 annual American Society of Anesthesiologists meeting (Shelley et al. 1993). A research grant was made by the APSF to continue the work displayed at the meeting (Schneider 1996). In 1994 the lab received the First Prize for Best Scientific Exhibit at the Annual ASA meeting (Mentzer 1994) and, more recently, has been awarded an "Excellence in Teaching" commendation by the problem-based learning classes of the Medical College.

4. COMMUNITY INVOLVEMENT

Since this report involves simulator involvement with learners other than traditional medical students, it seems appropriate to briefly describe some of the groups who have visited the lab. Primary school students, often visiting on career day or as part of community awareness programs, have been among the most enthusiastic guests. Grade school students are fascinated by the breathing plastic man and particularly interested in monitoring their own peripheral oxygen saturation, EKG or blood pressure. The education lab has been very well used by groups of Scouts, usually interested in either First Aid or Computer merit badges. Our community offers fairly complete convention accommodations and meeting groups have made arrangements to visit the lab. We provided members of the Pennsylvania State Society of Anesthesiologists with a simulator experience in geriatric anesthesia. A group of conventioning instrument engineers were just as interested in the wiring diagrams as the physiology.

Various groups of medical technicians have used the lab. Emergency room workers, personnel from our helicopter transport service, ambulance operators and paramedics have all had practical, hands-on, and usually recurring, courses. The ability to simulate airway problems, with real time changes in pulse oximeter readings, has been particularly helpful in training emergency care technicians.

5. HIGH SCHOOL SIMULATOR USE

Enthusiastic word of the capabilities of the simulator spread through our community to high school level curriculum planners who contacted the lab and asked for demonstrations of possible supplements to their science and health programs. Science, health, and physical education teachers from several local school districts made separate appointments for introductory visits. Most of the visitors were enthusiastic about the experience and asked to participate in joint projects.

One involved project was the Pennsylvania Youth Apprenticeship Program which is administered by both county government and two local school districts. At our end at the College of Medicine, most liaison work was done through the Department of Nursing. The teaching concept is the familiar one of exposing high school students to various opportunities for career development using the resources of the community. We believe that the ours is the only medical college to participate in such a program in Pennsylvania.

In this program, eleventh grade students who have expressed some interest in health related careers, spend two-week periods visiting various locations in the hospital such as nursing, dietetics, food preparation, administration and finance, clinics, etc. Visits to specialty clinical areas such as surgery, radiology, and anesthesiology are also included. A two hour visit to the education lab and an exploration of computer simulated normal physiology comprised the eleventh grade anesthesia experience.

During the senior year of high school, the students are permitted to choose two areas of special career interest and to spend portions of a semester in becoming more familiar with each. Course instructors define responsibilities and tasks for the students within the interest areas. The program carries course credits and has so far been limited to students with above average academic performance.

The major interaction has been with the eleventh grade students with a simulation not of anesthetized patients, but of fairly normal people undergoing physiological stresses of exercise and excitement. Formal educational goals for these encounters included stimulating an interest in science for the students and providing a different way to demonstrate aspects of health and wellness. Course instructors felt that they were participating in community outreach projects and stimulating interest and understanding in the activities of anesthesiologists.

6. SCENARIO OUTLINE

Simulator lab experiences were provided to small groups of high school students, two to three in an ideal group. The scenario presented to the students was that of two friends driving along a lonely country road and running out of gasoline. They decide to walk to the nearest farmhouse for a telephone and help. As they enter the farm yard a large dog chases them. One of the friends is a member of a marathon team and the other is accustomed to a sedentary and physically inactive lifestyle (couch potato.) Differences in the physiological response of each to the exercise were demonstrated with prearranged simulation programs.

7. SCENARIO MANAGEMENT

As a first step the high school students were introduced to the simulator and its component parts. The radial and carotid pulses were found, breath sounds were heard with stethoscopes, the heart was auscultated and the regular movement of the chest was pointed out. A question and answer format was used to determine and build on each student group's existing knowledge of physiology and normal values for vital signs. Some time was taken to practice these basic monitoring skills; students were individually coached.

The mannequin was actually monitored by a Hewlett Packard Merlin monitor which was capable of presenting far too many wave forms and too much data for an introductory experience. All monitoring channels were inactivated except those displaying the electrocardiogram, non-invasive blood pressure, heart rate, peripheral oxygen saturation, the capnogram and the respiratory rate. The students were familiarized with the data displays, which were helpfully of different colors. Capnogram and electrocardiogram waveforms were briefly described, no effort was made to include anything more than the most basic capnography and electrocardiogram interpretation. Interesting and challenging opportunities to ask and answer questions about what is being monitored, how it is being monitored, what the units of monitoring might be, what normal values might be, and how those values might normally vary were all presented. An interesting question was to ask the students why the blood pressure was measured in units of length rather than pressure (mmHg is, of course, not really a length measure.). Often a question about normal values was answered by having students monitor their own physiology.

7.1. The Athlete

The students were asked to predict the changes in vital signs that would occur when the marathon athlete was chased by a dog. Our subject began with a BP of 110/70 mmHg, a heart rate of 58 beats per minute and a respiratory rate of 11 breaths per minute. The simulator produced a blood pressure of 115/75 mmHg, heart rate of 68 and a respiratory rate of 14 when the athlete exercised by running.

7.2. The Sedentary Runner

After having been given baseline values for the athlete, and comparing them to their own baseline vital signs, the students were asked to decide what they believed the baseline vital signs of the sedentary runner might be. A typical set of predicted values might have been: blood pressure 140/87, heart rate 93 and respiratory rate of 17. The next predictions of vital signs, or at least predictions of the direction in which vital signs might change, were made for the exercising sedentary runner. The programmed changes produced by the simulator were: blood pressure 150/97, heart rate 100 and respiratory rate of 25.

The instructor then acted and demonstrated the running and sweating of the two anxious friends, and imitated the panting and out-of-breath sedentary runner. The simulator and monitor simultaneously displayed the heart and respiratory rates. The students usually became totally involved, not noticing from whence the information came—the instructor or the simulator. This "suspension of disbelief" seemed to be so complete that the students

Table 1. Questionnaire results. Eleventh grade
Pennsylvania Youth Apprenticeship students

	Yes	No
1. Is this a better way to learn science than books or lectures	17	0
2. Science taught with a human simulator is:		
Worse than books or lectures	0	
About the same as books and lectures	0	
Better than books and lectures	0	
Much better than books and lectures	17	0
3. Would you like to learn about other subjects with the simulator?	17	0
4. What might be good subjects for simulator learning:		
'Doctor patient relationships"	1	
"Basic surgical procedures"	2	
"Anatomy"	2	
"Information presented at the heart station"	1	
"Anesthesia"	2	
"How drugs affect the brain, drug abuse"	3	
"Changes of pregnancy"	2	
"Cardio-pulmonary resuscitation"	3	
"Biology"	1	
"Signs of illness"	1	
"Computer utilization"	1	
"Chemistry"	1	
5. Did the simulator raise questions you wanted to look up?	5	12
6. Did you actually look up answers to questions?	2	3
Medical books in library	1	
Computer	1	
7. Did you tell your friends about the simulator?	16	1
8. What was the best part of the simulator experience?		

"The dummy actually had vital signs"
"When we listened to the fake heart beats"
"Seeing the chest rise on a plastic body and feeling the pulse"
"How it actually portrayed a real patient"
"Seeing how your body reacts to different things"
"It was more realistic than just hearing from a preceptor"
"Different heart rates, how realistic it really was"
"Just seeing the simulator have a pulse and heartbeat like a normal person"
"Learning what anesthesiologists do"
"The realness of it"
"Seeing something so real-life that is completely man made"
"Being in a real-life experience"
"Working hands on with a patient who was not real and did not have feelings"
"Learning what the different lines on the monitor mean" (2 identical responses)
"Getting to listen to the heartbeats"
9. What was the worst part of the simulator experience?
"It is not a real person"
"I thought everything was interesting"
"Dwelling on one subject" (a pulse or heart rate)
"That the person (dummy) could not talk back, you can't ask questions"
"I got tired of standing" (2 responses)
"There was none" (10 responses)
No comment (1 response)

| 10. Do you think the simulator would be a good way to learn about street drugs? | 17 | 0 |

ignored the fact that the mannequin was lying supine on a table and was not running at all. It was very helpful to have an enthusiastic instructor, who was also somewhat of an amateur actor, to reach this level of involvement.

Again, the activities prompted many questions, some related to the simulation in action, others not related.

8. RESULTS

A questionnaire administered to the students demonstrated unanimous acceptance of the simulator as a valuable and interesting teaching tool. Several students made suggestions for expanding this form of teaching. The students were so impressed with the experience that several of the youth apprenticeship program students brought their science, health and physical education teachers with them on subsequent visits.

9. CONCLUSION

Using a full human simulator to complement science teaching for high school students has, in our opinion, been a huge success. We are planning to expand the program to demonstrate other physiological effects of other unhealthy lifestyles and to include alterations brought about by various types of substance abuse.

ACKNOWLEDGMENTS

We would like to thank Jody Henry for assistance with scenario development, data collection and preparartion of the figure.

REFERENCES

Mentzer S, Murray WB, Schneider AJL, Marshall WK, Shelley KH, Taekman J, Vaduva S, Foster PA, Roeckel M. Implementation of Cognitive Science in Anesthesiology Education and Training. Scientific Exhibit, ASA Annual Meeting (American Society of Anesthesiologists), San Francisco, CA, Oct 1994.

Murray WB, Foster PA, Schneider AJL, Robbins R. The new residents' first 3 days: measuring the efficacy of an introduction to clinical anesthesia with perceived self-efficacy. Research presentation , ASA Meeting, San Francisco, CA, Oct 1994.

Schneider AJL, Murray WB, Mentzer SC, Miranda F, Vaduva S. "Helper"—A critical events prompter for unexpected emergencies. Jnl Clin Mon 1995; 11 (6):358–364.

Shelley K, Schneider AJL, Mentzer S, Halm M. The use of interactive displays in Anesthesia. Scientific Exhibit, ASA Annual Meeting, Washington, DC, Oct 1993.

3

INTEGRATION OF THE HUMAN PATIENT SIMULATOR INTO THE MEDICAL STUDENT CURRICULUM

Life Support Skills

Eugene B. Freid

Department of Anesthesiology
University of North Carolina at Chapel Hill

To date, the main educational thrust of anesthesia (human patient) simulators has been on learning and practice in the operating room environment. The utility of anesthesia simulators in medical practice outside the operating room is just recently being realized. The human patient simulator has a number of attributes that make it useful in teaching, and possibly evaluating, the skills necessary to care for the acutely ill patient. As critical care itself developed as an extension of the operating room environment, the use of simulation in critical care education is an expected evolution of this technology.

In the United States, the medical student curriculum has been evolving into one of primary care and outpatient focus. The amount of time during their clinical education that medical students spend in acute, tertiary care, settings continues to decrease. In most medical schools, critical care topics are addressed in elective clerkships available to only a handful of students. It has become apparent to a number of critical care educators that the critical care education of medical students has been severely neglected[1]. The Society of Critical Care Medicine, concerned by the dearth of critical care education in the current medical school curriculum has charged a committee on medical student education to focus on this issue. Some medical schools have recognized this flaw in the curriculum and are reintroducing courses with an acute care focus into the curriculum. We describe the introduction of an anesthesia simulator-assisted critical care course in a medical school curriculum.

At the University of North Carolina the anesthesia simulator (Human Patient Simulator or HPS) is integrated into two courses that teach acute care and life support skills. The introductory course, Life Support Skills I, is a mandatory course for all third year medical students. It is a one week course in which the students learn advanced cardiac life support (ACLS) skills. Based on an extended ACLS curriculum, this course covers recognition, diagnosis, and therapy for life-threatening events. Arrhythmia recognition, airway management, cardioversion and defibrillation, intravenous access, and monitoring for

Simulators in Anesthesiology Education, edited by Henson and Lee.
Plenum Press, New York, 1998.

15

transport are basic concepts relevant to both generalists and specialists. The course combines didactic, laboratory, and HPS teaching of ACLS skills. The HPS is specifically utilized in teaching airway skills and in demonstrating pharmacologic manipulation of the circulation. Prior to our use of the HPS, the pharmacologic demonstration and resuscitation lab was performed using an anesthetized canine model. With the use of the HPS the animal lab is no longer necessary. This is a significant cost savings to the university and decreases the requirement for laboratory animals.

A second course, Life Supports Skills II (LSS II), makes more extensive use of the HPS and will be focused on in this paper. It is an optional course, also one week in duration during the third year curriculum and follows the LSS I week to initiate a 2 week continuum. One half of the third year medical school class can currently be accommodated in the 12 weeks that the course is offered. In its first year LSS II was fully subscribed. The goal of the course is to teach third year medical students the cognitive and technical skills crucial to effectively care for critically ill patients. The LSS II course focuses on patient stabilization and emergency department and intensive care unit management rather than initial life support skills. It offers a more extensive experience in invasive and non-invasive monitoring, advanced diagnosis and therapy, and crisis management.

The students are taught to collect and integrate historical data, the physical examination, and laboratory and monitoring information to develop a problem list and therapeutic plan.

The LSS 2 course has three distinct components designed to challenge students with varied learning preferences. The components include lecture-discussions, clinical experience in the operating room, and instructor-directed scenarios and demonstrations using the HPS. The faculty for this course are all members of the Department of Anesthesiology, but have a broad perspective appropriate for a course of this nature. Seven of the faculty members are board certified in a primary care specialty as well as anesthesiology. Five of the faculty members have had formal training in either surgical or pediatric critical care. Two course faculty have postgraduate training in respiratory physiology or pharmacology. This broad perspective is critical at the present time as the medical schools' focus is on primary care. A faculty with primary care training has the advantage of understanding the educational needs of students whether they are to choose careers as generalists or specialists. In addition, the expanded involvement of the Anesthesiology Department within the medical school is a benefit both to the medical school and the Anesthesiology Department.

During the course of the week there are eleven hours of core lecture-discussions. The lecture-discussion topics are shown in Table 1. A one-hour ventilator workshop follows the lecture on mechanical ventilation. The goal of the lectures is to stimulate and foster interactive discussion of problems. The general format for the core lectures is similar to the Fundamentals of Critical Care Support Course (FCCS) developed by the Society of Critical Care Medicine and is a critical care equivalent to Pediatric Advanced Life Support

Table 1. LSS 2 Lectures

Advance airway	Head trauma and coma
Respiratory monitoring	Trauma
Respiratory failure	Surgical stress and pain control
PA catheter/cardiac monitoring	Ethics in critical care
Hemodynamic turbulence	Toxicology
Sepsis and shock	

and the Advanced Trauma Life Support courses. The goal of this course, like FCCS, is to provide exposure of the basic principles of critical care to providers who have not had or do not plan on formal critical care training[2].

The students spend approximately twelve hours in the operating room area paired with an anesthesiology attending. There are several goals pursued in the students' operating room experience. There is an opportunity for the students to practice their intravenous access skills and learn arterial and central venous cannulation. It gives them an opportunity to practice airway management skills, e.g. bag valve mask ventilation, laryngoscopy and endotracheal intubation in a living subject rather than a mannequin. It also allows the students a chance to acquire an understanding of the preoperative evaluation process and to understand assuring readiness for surgery. The students observe the intraoperative management of both healthy and critically ill patients. They witness intraoperative physiologic alterations and their management, the pharmacology of neuromuscular blocking drugs and anesthetics, and learn about perioperative risk factors and pain management.

The last part of the course is a series of sessions utilizing the HPS and, based on student evaluations, is highly rated as a positive educational experience. We make heavy use of instructor-driven simulations and a team approach to patient management (Fig. 1). There are 4 HPS sessions, ranging from one to two and one-half hours in duration, in which the students develop skills in airway management, evaluate and manage pulmonary crises, evaluate and manage shock and hemodynamic compromise and provide initial hospital care for a trauma patient. During the scenarios the students are grouped into teams which include a team leader, airway/respiratory personnel, and personnel to act as consultants, attain intravenous access, perform procedures and administer drugs.

The airway management simulation on day 1 of the course provides an extension of the students basic airway skills. We demonstrate, and the students subsequently practice, blind nasal intubation in a spontaneous breathing patient, laryngeal mask airway (LMA) and esophageal-tracheal Combitube insertion, and retrograde wire techniques. Students

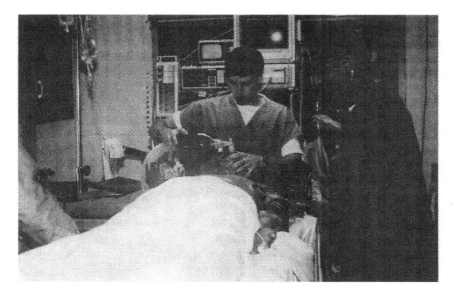

Figure 1. The team approach to management of a trauma patient.

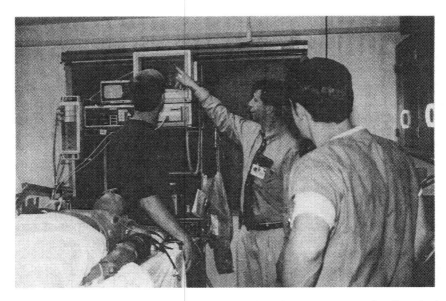

Figure 2. A system for analysis of hemodynamic data and pharmacologic management of cardiogenic shock is demonstrated.

learn needle cricothyrotomy and the use of jet ventilation during difficult airway sequences. A series of instructor-driven scenarios using a team approach to manage a series of airway problems follows. The scenarios include narcotic-induced apnea with difficult mask ventilation requiring the use of an oral airway, and several "can ventilate but cannot intubate" and "cannot ventilate, cannot intubate" scenarios. Scenarios with both spontaneously breathing and apneic subjects are presented.

On the third day of the course a simulator session is presented in which a series of pulmonary problems are managed again using a team approach. Problems include evaluation and management of mainstem intubation, bronchospasm, anaphylaxis, pneumothorax and adult respiratory distress syndrome. The techniques learned in the airway simulator session are integrated into these scenarios and the students build on information that they learn.

The fourth day of the course includes a two and one-half hour hemodynamic and shock session in which the students learn to evaluate and manage vasovagal syncope, hypovolemic and hemorrhagic shock, sepsis, anaphylactic shock, cardiac tamponade and neurogenic shock (Fig. 2). In some patients, respiratory distress is also present and the students learn to treat multiple system failure. There is a demonstration of the use pulmonary artery catheter and its role in pharmacologic strategies for the patient with cardiogenic shock. During this demonstration, the students observe the positive and negative attributes of fluids, inotropes, vasopressors, and vasodilators in the cardiogenic shock setting (Fig 3).

On the final day of the course is a one-hour "putting it all together" simulation. This scenario involves a patient who has been involved in a major automobile accident with multiple traumatic injuries (Fig. 4). The patient has a closed head injury with a basilar skull fracture, a left sided pneumothorax, pulmonary contusions and a fractured femur. Depending on the skill level of the students a difficult airway and a series of hemodynamic problems may also be introduced into the scenario.

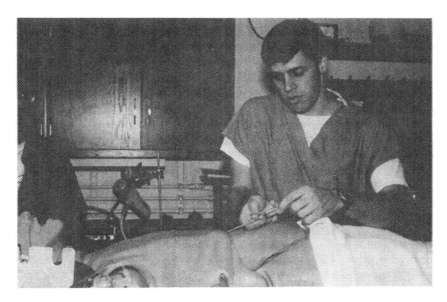

Figure 3. Learning pericardiocentesis in cardiac tamponade scenario.

At the end of the week there is a written exam designed to evaluate the students understanding of the material which also provides an indirect method of assessing the effectiveness of the course faculty. It includes multiple choice and short answer questions as well a question involving the evaluation and the development of an initial management plan for a complex critically ill patient. The students are also evaluated based on their per-

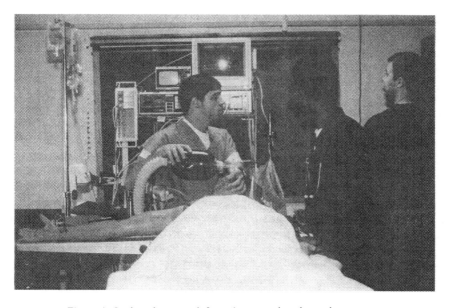

Figure 4. Students learn to ask for assistance and work together as a team.

formance in the lecture-discussions, operating room, and simulator lab. We currently have no formal mechanism to evaluate the students' performances during the patient simulator exercises. We are in the process of developing a scoring system for evaluating our anesthesiology residents during HPS exercises and would like to develop a similar system for evaluating the medical students. The HPS could be used in the place of a live patient model employed in the Objective Structured Clinical Exam (OSCE) method of evaluating critical care knowledge as described by Rogers[3].

The course is extensively evaluated by the students and the evaluations are confidentially sent to the medical school. The course has been very well accepted and the students especially enjoy the use of the HPS. Without fail, the students ask for more time in the HPS lab. We have found a number of advantages provided by the use of a simulator-assisted educational program. Most importantly the simulator offers a '"hands on", "real time" and repeatable system. The students are challenged to compile historical information, extract data from serial examinations of the mannequin and to develop a problem list and treatment priorities. The students learn to examine repetitively and observe for changes in the status of the simulated patient. It is one the few times during the third year of medical school that the students actually are able to make decisions based on their own evaluation. It allows them to integrate a clinical history, their own senses and monitoring data to develop a problem list and treatment plan not usually possible during their third year clerkships. The students develop an understanding of triage and crisis management. They learn to work with their peers as part of a team rather than as an individual unlike most of their preceding course work in medical school. It also gives the students a sense of immediate gratification, the fact they can solve problems and take care of patients with a positive outcome.

There are several problems with using the HPS in this course that provide stumbling blocks to achieving a truly realistic experience. One significant problem is the lack of central nervous system reality. The student's inability to evaluate the level of consciousness, examine deep tendon reflexes and pupillary signs is a shortcoming of the technology. In the simulations the instructor must tell the students what neurologic signs and symptoms are present. A second problem with the simulator technology are the mechanical sounds that give clues not present in the clinical scenario. Mechanical sounds of respiration can obviate the need for chest auscultation. Other mechanical sound include the sounds of the pulse and sometimes the inflation of the airway obstruction apparatus. The instructor must avoid cues which can tip the students to upcoming changes in patient status as well and must be avoided.

One difficulty with a course of this nature is the significant variability in the clinical acumen of the students over the course of the year. The early groups have just completed their second year of medical school and they have a limited clinical experience from which to draw on. It is impressive how rapidly the students learn the evaluation skills and ask the appropriate questions to be able to solve the problems using their basic science knowledge. Early in the week the students react slowly, but as the week goes on the students skills in evaluation and management improve rapidly. Later in the year as the students have a broader clinical base, we can make the scenarios more complicated. Individual students can also have the scenarios adjusted to their clinical level so as to always push them. The students have found the course material intellectually challenging, but none of the students have felt that the course material is overwhelming.

Our initial use of the patient simulator suggests that the use of simulator-assisted education may provide a means to assess the student's skills. A format for effectively assessing the medical students critical care skills has been a problem for the medical schools in which critical care education is part of their curriculum. An accurate and non biased mechanism to effectively assess the students ability to evaluate and manage the acutely ill patient is currently lacking. Several institutions use written exams however the written exam does not assess the students examination and integration skills[4]. The use of the OSCE format is appealing but requires the use of a "live" patient simulation which precludes allowing the student to actually administer therapy. The use of the HPS for the assessment of medical students critical care skills has not yet been described, but is likely to occur in the near future. In our judgment the use of the HPS provides an excellent format for teaching critical care skills . The current technology is associated with some minor pitfalls which small compared to the advantages that the technology offers.

REFERENCES

1. Buchman TG, Dellinger RP, Raphaely RC, Todres ID. Undergraduate education in critical care medicine. Critical Care Medicine, 1992; 20: 1595–1603.
2. Dellinger RP. Fundamentals of Critical Care Support: Another merit badge or more? Critical Care Medicine, 1996; 556–557.
3. Rogers P, Jacob H, Thomas E, Willenkin R. Objective structured clinical examinations (OSCE) demonstrate improved thinking and application skills after a critical care medicine (CCM) elective. Critical Care Medicine, 1996 24:S45.
4. Rogers PL, Grenvik A, Willenkin RL. Teaching medical students complex cognitive skills in the intensive care unit. Critical Care Medicine, 1995 23:575–581.

4

USING SIMULATORS FOR MEDICAL STUDENTS AND ANESTHESIA RESIDENT EDUCATION

Andrew C. Lee

Department of Anesthesiology
University of Rochester School of Medicine
Rochester, New York

1. INTRODUCTION

Over the last several years, there has been a dramatic increase in the use of anesthesia human patient simulators for educational purposes. Full-scale, computer run simulators are currently being used to teach courses ranging from basic instruction of non-anesthesiologists to the more complicated Anesthesia Crisis Resource Management[TM,1] for continuing medical education of attending anesthesiologists. At the University of Rochester, the emphasis of our simulator program has been in the education of medical students and anesthesia residents. This chapter will not only provide an outline of the different courses for which we have used the simulator as an educational adjunct, but also to share some of the lessons we have learned that will help in creating a successful educational program.

Although education using 3-dimensional anesthesia simulators is a relatively new field, it seems to have many potential benefits. The value of simulators in medical education lies in the ability to create a "standard patient" for operator-controlled situations. For teaching basic science courses such as physiology or pharmacology, the simulated patient can reliably reproduce whatever clinical situation the facilitator intends. These scenarios can be repeated with several groups of students as needed. Different physiologic parameters can be augmented to make teaching points more dramatic. Because the preclinical students have little experience with patient contact, this clinical emphasis helps increase interest and attention. For more clinical-based teaching, the simulator allows facilitators and users to examine and improve clinical decision making processes and to practice specific clinical scenarios or crises. Practice on the simulator should make the user more comfortable and knowledgeable when faced with the same "live" clinical situations. The impact of simulator training on patient outcome, however, has been difficult to objectively quantify for several reasons: there is an overwhelming number of confounding variables, the crises are extremely infrequent, and objective evaluation of practitioners in a real crisis situation is difficult to perform. There have been several studies[2] undertaken to evalu-

Simulators in Anesthesiology Education, edited by Henson and Lee.
Plenum Press, New York, 1998.

ate benefit, but solid rigorous evidence is still lacking. Because of the high cost of anesthesia simulators in terms of financial resources and non-clinical hours, studies confirming the benefits of simulators in education may be necessary before the value of this educational tool has widespread acceptance.

2. MEDICAL STUDENT PROGRAMS

2.1. Introduction

At the University of Rochester, we are integrating the anesthesia simulator into several areas of our educational program. Currently, the emphasis of the simulator educational program is on medical student and resident education. For the junior medical students, the simulator is used to teach subjects that are difficult to understand without a "live" clinical correlation. Specific teaching objectives are identified and scenarios can be chosen to dramatically demonstrate those objectives. This can be done without live patient's being subjected to one hundred first or second year medical students standing at their bedside. The simulator can be brought into the lecture halls or the students can come to the simulator educational area in smaller groups for seminar-like sessions. For the senior medical students, training with the anesthesia simulator allows them to develop more confidence in clinical patient care. They are confronted with a clinical problem in which they must create a differential diagnosis, develop a treatment plan, carry it out, and see the results of their actions without an attending or resident physician dictating their decisions. The students are able to practice and develop their clinical decision making skills, independently or in small groups, in a way that does not put real patients at risk. This type of training will never supplant a medical education system that involves live patients but it appears to be a valuable adjunct. The goal of the medical student educational programs is not to specifically teach the specialty of "anesthesiology", but to focus on decision making skills, procedures and theory that can carry through any area of medicine that they might pursue.

2.2. Preclinical Section

The medical student simulator education programs are divided into preclinical and clinical sections. The Department of Anesthesiology is involved in teaching the respiratory physiology course to the first year medical student class. We looked to see if there was a part of this lecture series that would benefit from the anesthesia human patient simulator; specifically, we were looking for topics within respiratory physiology that were difficult to learn or understand with the traditional didactic method or seminars. We decided that the concepts of pulmonary compliance and resistance and their associated pressure volume curves would benefit from a lecture with "live" demonstration using the simulator. The simulator was moved to the first year medical student lecture hall. A camera, aimed at the analog pressure-volume displays of an anesthesia machine, projected them in real-time onto a large screen in front of the students. A specialist in respiratory physiology then proceeded with a lecture about pulmonary resistance and compliance. With a simulated intubated patient, peak and plateau pressures were described. Using the simulator it was possible to clearly explain the principles of resistance and compliance that are usually very confusing when using static images. Once the description was made, a clinical scenario was used to complete the educational exercise. A trauma patient with a history of asthma was simulated to make these demonstrations even more complete. Changes in pulmonary compliance and resistance were seen in a "real" case so that the clinical correlation could be made. Immediate feedback from the students was overwhelmingly positive.

There is one other preclinical simulator-based course that was designed this year. The purpose of this course was to create an alternative for medical students who did not want to participate in the pharmacology animal laboratory. We designed this course to cover the same pharmacologic interventions that were to be reviewed in a living cat laboratory, but to involve the anesthesia human patient simulator as the subject. We reviewed a variety of sympathomimetic agents, muscarinic and nicotinic agonists as well as several alpha, beta and cholinergic antagonists. This course was done in an interactive question-discussion format with small groups of seven or less students. Immediate feedback from this course has already been positive and our plans are to continue offering this alternative.

2.3. Clinical Section

The *clinical* courses set up for the medical students include sections of the General Clerkship course (which is an introduction to clinical medicine at the beginning of the third year of medical school), Perioperative Medicine (designed and offered by the Department of Anesthesiology) and the Anesthesia Clerkship.

2.3.1. General Clerkship. As a part of their pre-clinical General Clerkship, third year medical students are given a course on basic airway and pain management by the Department of Anesthesiology. A session with the simulator integrates the didactic parts of this course into a clinical scenario. The instructors provide an introduction to the simulator and then facilitate a scenario that simulates a patient who has been given an opioid overdose in the postoperative period. Topics covered during the simulation include treatment of postoperative pain, control of ventilation, side effects of opioids, and management of the unconscious and apneic patient. The entire medical student class is divided into groups of 5–8 people and the scenarios are repeated over the course of several days. This course is designed to begin the difficult integration process of didactic knowledge and clinical skills.

2.3.2. Anesthesiology Clerkship. Third year and fourth year medical students in the Anesthesiology Clerkship take part in two sessions with the simulator; an introductory course and a wrap-up session. The introductory session, which follows a basic airway management course, is designed to introduce the students to the operating room from the anesthesiologist's point of view. They are taught the basics of the anesthesia machine, physiologic monitoring and routine induction of anesthesia and airway management. This session is meant to ease the transition into the operating room environment and get the students up to speed as to what is going on from the first day. This session was added at previous students' request. They felt that too much of their rotation was spent deciphering the mystery of the anesthesia machine and monitors. At the end of their clerkship, the students have another session with the anesthesia simulator. This session involves a more clinically advanced situation which includes such areas as; induction of general anesthesia, intubation, and management of a critical incident such as massive blood loss. A difficult intubation scenario is also reviewed. The students make all of the clinical decisions independently and are able to see the immediate results. This session is performed in a non-threatening, non-test environment which allows the students to integrate what they have learned during the rotation, as well as display those skills. In other words, this final session acts as an excellent conclusion or debriefing of the overall elective. Both simulator sessions have been positively reviewed by the students.

2.3.3. Perioperative Medicine. The Department of Anesthesiology also offers a course in Perioperative Medicine to third and fourth year medical students. This course is designed to introduce students to the idea of anesthesiologists are perioperative doctors. The simulator is used to teach some sections of perioperative care including hemodynamic monitoring, intraoperative complications and basic crisis management. We decided that these topics could be adequately covered in a more time efficient manner using the simulator rather than the students rotating through actual cases in the operating room. The instructors were able to spend more time teaching the specific topics to this group of students, rather than being distracted with patient care. The students did spend some time in the operating room, following assigned patients from preoperative evaluation, through the intraoperative period, and to the postoperative period and discharge. The simulator sessions did not take away from actual patient contact. In fact, it probably made the time spent in the operating room more efficient in learning other aspects of perioperative care. The simulator sessions, as well as the overall course, has been received very positively by the students.

2.4. Medical Student Programs: Conclusion

As you can see from the summary of these programs, there are many benefits of running simulator based medical student teaching programs. These benefits apply not only to the students themselves, but to the department that is running the simulator programs. These include:

- The ability to bring *clinical applicability* to the early medical students.
- The ability to teach topics that are difficult to teach in a purely didactic form.
- The provision of a natural bridge between didactic and clinical work that is safe.
- An introduction to our specialty and our department early in a student's career.
- An ability to provide a service that increases our standing in the local and national medical community.

3. ANESTHESIA RESIDENT PROGRAMS

3.1. Introduction to Clinical Anesthesia

The anesthesia Human Patient Simulator is also used for the teaching of anesthesia residents at the University of Rochester. Early in their CA-1 year, anesthesia residents take part in a simulator course that is an Introduction to Clinical Anesthesia. This provides an introduction to anesthesia equipment, setup and the basics of induction of general anesthesia and intubation. The objectives of this course are to:

- Familiarize the new residents to the operating room environment
- Increase the speed and efficiency with setup and preparation
- Increase the comfort level with the routine of the administration of a general anesthetic.

The use of checklists, videotaping and debriefing are all used to improve the learning process and to let the residents see themselves at work. Videotaping and debriefing are essential components of the experience as this allows the residents to see themselves performing tasks within a given system. Viewing oneself and debriefing the session are powerful educational tools that come to the anesthesia simulator program from aviation cockpit training programs and was assimilated to anesthesia human patient simulators by Dr. David Gaba in his Anesthesia Crisis Resource Management (ACRM) program[1,3,4]. This technique has also been adopted by other training groups involving trauma resuscitation, et cetera.

3.2. Advanced Clinical Scenarios

Later in their training the anesthesia residents are introduced to more complex clinical scenarios (such as the management of cardiac tamponade, malignant hyperthermia, difficult airways, abdominal aortic aneurysm clamping and unclamping, changes in airway compliance, etc.) as well as some more technically oriented ones (machine fault workshop, line isolation monitor, jet ventilation). The objective of these courses is to introduce and practice approaches to "low frequency" clinical situations. It is important to suit the scenario with the resident's level of experience and to move them through a teaching program progressively. These courses are taught daily, from 7–7:45 a.m. with the resident assigned to the preoperative clinic or the postanesthesia care unit.

3.3. Difficult Airway Course

Finally, the simulator is used to teach a section of the Difficult Airway Course which is offered to anesthesia residents and nurse anesthetists four times per year. The simulator session begins with a review of the American Society of Anesthesiologists (ASA) Difficult Airway Algorithm, then two scenarios are used to practice different limbs of the algorithm: cannot intubate, can ventilate and cannot intubate cannot ventilate. This exercise allows the students to develop a plan for dealing with difficult airways and test it out in a life-like operating room situation. Although the exercise includes several technically oriented procedures, such as the performance of cricothyrotomy and the institution of transtracheal jet ventilation, the focus remains on decision making, resource management, communication and the ASA Difficult Airway Algorithm.

4. CONCLUSION

The human patient simulator education program at the University of Rochester has, so far, focused mainly on educating medical students and residents. Above is a summary of the courses which we have offered. We are continuing to offer more courses throughout the entire medical school curriculum, and are expanding our resident education program. Future ideas may involve multidisciplinary instruction in both the medical school and the residencies of the institution as well as the more organized and involved crisis resource management. The variety of courses that can be offered seems to be limited only by time constraints of the instructors and the imagination.

REFERENCES

1. Gaba DG, Fish KJ, Howard SK: Anesthesia Crisis Management. Churchill Livingston, 1994.
2. Chopra V, Gesink BJ, De Jong J, Bovill JG, Spierdijk J, Brand R: Does training on an anaesthesia simulator lead to improvement in performance? British Journal of Anaesthesia 73: 293, 1994.
3. Boston Anesthesia Simulation Center Anesthesia Crisis Resource Management Syllabus, Copyright 1994.
4. Helmreich RL, Chidester TR, Foushee HC, Gregorich S, Wilhelm JA: How Effective is Cockpit Resource Management Training? Flight Safety Foundation- Flight Safety Digest, May 1990.

OTHER RECOMMENDED READING

1. Cooper JB, Newbower RS, Kitz RJ: An Analysis of Major Errors and Equipment Failures in Anesthesia Management: Considerations for Prevention and Detection. Anesthesiology 60: 34, 1984.
2. Cooper JB, Gaba DM: A strategy for Preventing Anesthesia Accidents. International Anesthesiology Clinics 27: 148, 1989.
3. Cooper JB, Newbower RS, Long CD, McPeek B: Preventable Anesthesia Mishaps: A Study of Human Factors. Anesthesiology 49: 399, 1978.
4. Euliano T, Society for Education in Anesthesia 1995 Workshop: How to Use simulators for Medical Students and Residents.
5. Good M, Gravenstein J: Anesthesia simulators and Training Devices. International Anesthesiology Clinics 27: 161, 1989.
6. Howard SK, Gaba DM, Fish KJ, Yang G, Sarnquist FH: Anesthesia Crisis Resource Management Training: Teaching Anesthesiologists to Handle Critical Incidents. Aviation, Space, and Environmental Medicine 63: 763–770, 1992.

5

SIMULATION IN NURSING ANESTHESIA EDUCATION

Practical and Conceptual Perspectives

Alfred E. Lupien

Medical College of Georgia
Augusta, Georgia 30912

1. INTRODUCTION

Anesthesia care in the United States is delivered predominantly by physician anesthesiologists and nurse anesthetists. Approximately 22,000 nurse anesthetists represent 40%-50% of the actively practicing anesthesia providers in the United States.[1,2] The scope of practice for nurse anesthetists, as described by the American Association of Nurse Anesthetists, includes a complete range of services including pre-anesthetic evaluation, development of anesthesia plans, administration of general and regional anesthesia, and provision of post-anesthesia care.[3] Actual activities of nurse anesthetists vary from assistive roles to independent practice arrangements. Most commonly, nurse anesthetists work together with anesthesiologists in anesthesia care teams. Nurse anesthetists are the sole anesthesia providers for 20–25% of the American public and may provide as much as 65–85% of the anesthesia care in rural settings.[4,5,6]

The educational process for anesthetists differs from that of anesthesiologists. Admission to a nursing anesthesia program requires the student be a registered nurse, hold a bachelor's degree, and have at least one year of critical-care nursing experience.[7] Anesthesia programs are a minimum of 24 months in length, although the average length of a program is 27–28 months.[8] Most programs award a master's degree to graduates. The minimum time period for education following secondary education for nurse anesthetists is seven years compared to 12 years for anesthesiologists.[4] Although there are differences in educational preparation of nurse anesthetists and anesthesiologists, there is a universal standard of care.[9]

Since nursing anesthesia programs have a shorter duration of instruction, it is imperative that the educational processes for nurse anesthetists become efficient. Because simulation can play a significant role in optimizing education for anesthesia care providers, we have incorporated simulation into the Nursing Anesthesia Program at the Medical College of Georgia. Before I describe how we are using simulation from both practical and conceptual perspectives, additional background on the education of nurse anesthetists might be helpful.

Simulators in Anesthesiology Education, edited by Henson and Lee.
Plenum Press, New York, 1998.

2. OVERVIEW OF NURSING ANESTHESIA EDUCATION

Requirements for graduation from a nursing anesthesia program include completion of a minimum of 135 instructional hours in anatomy, physiology, and pathophysiology; 90 hours pharmacology; 90 hours practice priniciples; and 45 hours chemistry, biochemistry and physics. Students administer a minimum of 450 anesthetics in predetermined surgical categories using various anesthetic agents and techniques for general and regional anesthesia. Proficiency in technical skills such as endotracheal intubation and venous and arterial cannulation must be demonstrated.[7] Upon completion of the program, graduates are eligible to take a national certification examination administered by the Council on Certification of Nurse Anesthetists.

Educational programs for nurse anesthetists may be organized in a variety of curricular formats as along as the program complies with the Standards and Guidelines of the Council on Accreditation of Nurse Anesthesia Educational Programs. In general, curricula can be classified as either integrated or "front-loaded." Integrated programs mix classroom instruction with clinical practice throughout the program. The principal advantage of an integrated curriculum is the opportunity to reinforce students' classroom knowledge with immediate clinical application. Front-loaded programs provide a 9–12 month foundation in basic science and anesthesia principles before concentrated clinical practice.[10] Front-loading also is used to conserve faculty costs by concentrating classroom instruction to central locations prior to students entering into a clinical residency which may be distant from the academic institution.[11]

3. AN EXAMPLE OF SIMULATOR USE IN NURSING ANESTHESIA EDUCATION

The Medical College of Georgia began an educational program for nurse anesthetists in September, 1995. The program uses a front-loaded curricular model which can be divided into three overlapping phases with distinct goals, implementation strategies, and intended outcomes. At the time of this presentation, we have implemented only the first two phases of the program. The final phase will be implemented in the upcoming months.

3.1. Phase I: Pre-Clinical Education

The pre-clinical phase of the program provides students a basis for initial learning and continued growth as anesthesia care providers. General goals are to establish a foundation in basic science from which to build further instruction in anesthesia-related topics and to introduce anesthesia management principles commonly used by nurse anesthetists. Coursework includes anatomy, physiology, pathophysiology, and pharmacology. Simulation is used in lieu of animal laboratory sessions to illustrate principles of cardiovascular and respiratory function. Session topics include hemodynamics and cardiovascular function, cardiovascular pharmacology, respiratory dynamics and pulmonary function, and positive pressure ventilation.

Since experience in high acuity nursing is a requisite for admission to the anesthesia program, students have experience with many of the clinical tools used in the diagnosis and/or management of cardiopulmonary responses. The simulation sessions are intended to establish a uniform base of experiences from which to continue in the educational process and assure a sound conceptual base to compliment practical experience.

Simulation is also used to introduce the clinical activities of the nurse anesthetist. Students are oriented to the Anesthesia Simulation Laboratory and the common features of anesthesia equipment and monitoring systems. Basic procedures are demonstrated such as regional anesthesia techniques and administration of general anesthesia from induction through maintenance and emergence. In addition to technical skills, some of the more tacit aspects of anesthesia care are illustrated such as the safety mechanisms integrated into an anesthesia machine.

One of the more dramatic introductory simulation sessions features two induction sequences intended to emphasize the importance of anesthesia care planning and decision making. The first induction sequence appears to be routine. Thiopental and succinylcholine are administered to a standard patient. The fundamental actions of the drugs are described. The instructor comments that these short-acting agents have been selected because their effects will terminate before hypoxic damage occurs if ventilation can not be established. The instructor does not ventilate the simulator, symbolizing an inability to ventilate despite all efforts. Students are asked to predict the outcome. If the hypothesis is true, that the drug effects will terminate before an untoward event occurs, then the simulator will resuscitate itself. As the discussion continues hypercarbia and hypoxemia ensue. The simulated patient ultimately sustains a cardiac arrest.

Students are asked to suggest ways to modify the induction sequence to safeguard the patient against poor outcomes. The concept of preoxygenation is discussed and the induction sequence if repeated after the simulator has been preoxygenated. As in the first scenario, the provider is unable to ventilate the patient following succinylcholine administration; however, oxygen reserve is sufficient and succinylcholine-induced paralysis terminates prior to cardiac arrest. Spontaneous ventilation is restored without practitioner intervention. While the demonstration may be characterized as overly dramatic and contrived, it is a useful example of how simulation can illustrate care planning and decision making to individuals with minimal anesthesia experience.

In addition to anesthesia-related topics, students participate in a series of nursing courses including theoretical models for nursing practice, health care issues, and research. In each of the classes, students are expected to relate course content to their field of practice. Since students have no experience with the delivery of anesthesia, simulation experiences are combined with classroom activities and self-directed reading to introduce students to the role of anesthesia care providers.

At the completion of the first phase of instruction, students possess a set of common experiences from which to build the remainder of their anesthesia education. The base includes a common vocabulary, an appreciation for concepts that are significant for anesthesia practice, and a framework for building a comprehensive education in anesthesia.

3.2. Phase II: The Transition to Clinical Practice

The second phase of the curriculum focuses on anesthesia-specific content. Topics of instruction include applied organic and biochemistry, physics, anesthesia pharmacology, and fundamentals of practice. The purpose of this phase of instruction is to prepare students for clinical practice.

The anesthesia simulator is used extensively as students participate in bi-weekly laboratory sessions for 12 weeks. Anesthesia practice techniques are refined from isolated tasks into sequences of action. The development of airway management skills illustrates the building process. During early sessions, basic techniques of airway management; such as insertion of pharyngeal airways, endotracheal intubation, and needle cricothyroidotomy; are taught and practiced. As the student progresses, the isolated tasks are incorporated into a schema for airway management which integrates technical skills with a process for decision-making. The management of various "ventilate but can't intubate" and "can't ventilate-can't intubate" scenarios are practiced based on defined strategies for airway management such as the ASA Difficult Airway Algorithm. Ultimately, the concept of airway management is integrated into complete sequences for the induction of general anesthesia. To prepare students for clinical practice, instructors mimic teaching strategies which are commonly used in the operating room. During the simulation exercises, the student's progress through a sequence of actions may be interrupted for clarification of medication doses, rationale for action, and discussions about alternative management strategies.

The development of good clinical decision making and technical skills are emphasized during training sessions. Manual skills are closely supervised by faculty working with groups of up to six individuals. Within each group, students work in pairs so that while one student is practicing a skill, the second student can reinforce comments of the instructor, provide feedback, and learn vicariously. Once the student has demonstrated minimal competency in the required technical skills, the focus of teaching shifts from skills acquisition to decision making. A process for clinical decision making is modeled by the faculty. As the sessions progress, responsibility for decision making shifts from faculty to the student. When unanticipated events develop, students are expected to evaluate the situation, consider possible courses of action, implement a plan, evaluate the effectiveness of the selection, and manage consequences as needed.

Practical testing is an integral part of the simulation exercises. Preliminary examinations focus on isolated skills in airway management and techniques for the administration of subarachnoid and epidural anesthesia. The final examination includes the management of a routine induction. Integrated action and critical thought processes are evaluated. If unanticipated events occur, the student is expected to manage the events as they arise.

The purpose of testing is twofold. First, it serves as a mechanism to assure that students have the appropriate technical and decision making skills to progress to the clinical portion of the program. Second, it prepares the students for practice in clinical settings where each of their actions will be closely scrutinized and evaluated.

Unsupervised simulator practice is encouraged to augment the supervised sessions. The primary focus of the unsupervised sessions is refinement of skills introduced in supervised sessions. Students work together in small groups and can use the simulation laboratory as frequently as they desire. Handouts detailing procedures, such as induction sequences, are provided by the faculty. Textbooks, such as Crisis Management in Anesthesiology (Gaba DM, Fish KJ, Howard, SK: Crisis Management in Anesthesiology. New York, Churchill Livingstone, 1994), are used by the students as supplemental references. The simulation laboratory is located adjacent to the faculty offices to assure the availability of an instructor for consultation and to monitor appropriate use of the simulator and associated equipment.

Intended outcomes of the pre-clinical phase of the program include familiarity and experience with basic induction sequences and the management of common anesthesia problems. Each student completes 20–30 induction sequences in the simulation laboratory prior to administering their first anesthetic to a living patient. Since many of the teaching strategies used during simulation sessions mimic actual intra-theater strategies, it is hoped that students are more prepared for what to expect once they begin practice in the operating room. Ideally, the students' familiarity with the management of tasks will allow them to look beyond the technical skills they are attempting to master and focus on the patient care that is being delivered.

Evaluation of the efficacy of our pre-clinical use of simulation is limited by the newness of our educational program. There are no previous classes of students for comparison. Informally, both students and faculty have reported that the students have been well-prepared for their initial clinical experiences. Written comments on daily clinical evaluations from preceptors accustomed to working with students from other programs suggest that the students are performing as well as, or better than, anticipated for their level of experience. Beginning students have demonstrated the ability to initiate and complete the technical aspects of routine induction sequences in an organized fashion to the satisfaction of their clinical preceptors.

3.3. Phase III: Clinical Phase

The final phase of the education program focuses on clinical performance and advanced topics in anesthesia practice. The underlying principles include reflective practice, critical thinking, and decision making.

As we implement the third phase of the program, the anesthesia simulation lab will be used in two ways. To promote continued development of students as practitioners, progressively complex scenarios are planned incorporating patient pathophysiology and the management of situations such as aortic clamping and unclamping. Students will experience uncommon events such as malignant hyperthermia, pneumothorax, and pericardial tamponade. It is anticipated that as scenarios increase in complexity, the focus of sessions will shift from solo management of anesthetics to effective utilization of anesthesia care teams and other resources.

The second use of the simulator will be to recreate situations as experienced by the students in the operating room. Students will be encouraged to reflect on the actual care provided, develop alternative treatments, and test the efficacy of the revised plans.

Intended outcomes of the final phase of the educational program include individual competency in the management of routine anesthesia care and common anesthesia problems, understanding of personal strengths and weakness as care providers, an appreciation for contributions of physician anesthesiologists and other health care colleagues to the anesthesia care team, and the development of strategies for critical thinking and refection in anesthesia practice.

4. LESSONS LEARNED

At this point in time, we consider ourselves novice users of an anesthesia simulator as we continue to accrue experiences. Based on our initial experiences with simulation, the following observations are offered.

4.1. Externalization of Thought

Students are encouraged to "think out loud" during simulation sessions. Speaking aloud has practical and conceptual advantages. Practically, it allows the instructor to monitor the simulation instead of becoming an artificial participant in the event a student's action goes unnoticed. The scenario is more natural if the participant makes informative general statements, such as "I'm giving 5 ml of succinylcholine," rather than directing conversation to the instructor-operator.

Conceptually, speech and thought are believed to be linked inextricably. The ability to communicate effectively is required for higher levels of cognitive development.[12] Encouraging the student to speak aloud acts as a "window to the mind" providing insight into the thought processes of the student. The instructor has an opportunity to monitor the student's perspective during a clinical situation. For example, when faced with hypotension and tachycardia following an uneventful induction of general anesthesia, the student may say, "I see that the blood pressure has dropped to 80/50, and heart rate has increased to 115. These changes are most likely caused by a relative hypovolemia from either being NPO overnight, or the vasodilation from isoflurane, or both. I think I'll decrease the concentration of isoflurane and increase the IV flow rate." The statement details what the student has observed, the differential diagnosis, and plan for action. The instructor is able to use the student's comments to determine whether all relevant information has been identified and used to develop the correct action plan. Potentially, the same process of thinking aloud may be used in the operating room to facilitate communication between a student and instructor.

4.2. Teaching Effectiveness

Simulation is also helpful in the evaluation of classroom instruction. The goal of didactic teaching in anesthesia education is to prepare students for clinical practice. Information should be presented in a fashion that is clinically useful. Ultimately, the operating theater becomes the optimal location for the evaluation of instruction. The generalizability of clinical evaluation of didactic instruction is limited by the inability to standardize the clinical situation for uniform evaluation of all students. Even if similar actual anesthesia scenarios can be constructed, student maturation as care providers can not be controlled as specific anesthesia content is acquired uniquely by each student based on the clinical situations encountered prior to evaluation.

Simulators provide a unique opportunity to standardize content so that each student can be exposed an identical situation over a limited time period (to minimize the effect of maturation). During a recent testing session, I had the opportunity to experience two events that highlight the use of anesthesia simulators tools for the evaluation of instruction.

Beginning students were asked to perform a routine induction on a healthy patient and initiate anesthesia maintenance. Following uneventful inductions, five of the six students introduced isoflurane for anesthesia maintenance by carefully "dialing in" 1 MAC of the agent. The sixth student initiated isoflurane at 2% but could provide no rationale for the decision. When asked to state the MAC of isoflurane, the student hesitated and stumbled before providing the correct answer. From the context of the interaction, I concluded that the decision to initiate the anesthetic with 2% isoflurane was not directly related to any objective criteria. I was surprised by the apparent lack of understanding of the uptake of inhalation anesthetics from all six students. Afterwards, the pharmacology instructor assured me that theoretical and practical aspects of uptake and distribution were discussed in great detail in the classroom and then illustrated using Gas Man® interactive software (Med Man Simulations, Inc., P.O. Box 67-160, Chestnut Hill, MA 02167, USA). The instructor agreed that students should have initiated isoflurane at a concentration greater than 1 MAC. For whatever reason, the didactic content did not transfer to present simulation.

We have also experienced the opposite phenomenon, where content taught within the context of simulation has not transferred to traditional pencil-and-paper testing. Over the course of a 12-week period, students were taught in the classroom about the concepts of preoxygenation and denitrogenation. In simulation sessions, a respiratory gas analyzer was used to determine objective end-point for pre-oxygenation (end-tidal $O_2 > 90\%$) rather than an arbitrary length of time. During the simulation testing sessions, each of the students used the appropriate clinical end-point to determine when preoxygenation was complete. The following day, during a traditional testing session, students uniformly wrote about preoxygenation "for two minutes" (which was not discussed in class but described by Willenkin RL, Polk SL: Management of general anesthesia, Anesthesia, 4th ed. Edited by Miller RD. New York, Churchill Livingstone, 1994, p 1050). For whatever reason, the clinical endpoint emphasized in the laboratory setting was not reiterated in the classroom setting.

5. EDUCATIONAL THEORY

In 1989, Brown, Collins, and Duguid coined the term situated cognition to describe their belief that learning can not separated from the activities that produced the learning.[13] They criticized traditional education systems that separated "knowing" from "doing." Their modern theory invokes a classical apprenticeship model where novice and expert work side by side in authentic activities. The learner constructs a new version of reality based on the activities being taught, the particular setting in which it is being taught, and his/her previous experience. Unlike the classical model of apprenticeship, the situated cognition model extends beyond the traditional focus on technical skills and includes the cognitive aspects typically associated with formal schooling. Although the term is new, the concept of situated cognition describes the system of cognitive apprenticeship that has been used for centuries in medical education.

Critics of the situated learning model argue that beginning education should be conducted in controlled settings.[14] Without the support of classroom experiences, students immersed in a practice setting will develop a set of skills limited by the situations encountered. Unless the teacher acts as a master, and exposes the student to expert conduct in a wide variety of settings, the apprenticeship will be incomplete.

Artificial situations, such as simulation also have been characterized as being "inauthentic" compared to real activities because learning through errors is encouraged. The consequences of actions in the simulated environment are less consequential that the consequences of real actions where error-free performance is expected.[15] One method for assessing consequences of actions in the simulation laboratory has been the administration of practical examinations with grading of performance. While the consequences of a poor test score can not be compared to the real-life implications of clinical practice, evaluation and testing add impetus for error-free performance. The use of simulation in nursing anesthesia education may be more life-like than in many other academic settings. As experienced critical care nurses, students bring to the simulation an appreciation of the implications of many of the simulated cardiovascular and respiratory events that occur. For anesthesia students and practitioners, the simulated environment may be uncomfortably realistic.

The design of our program embraces the situated cognition model while also responding to its primary criticism. In the early portions of the program, classroom instruction provides fundamental concepts and serves as an advanced organizer for future study.[16] The didactic instruction is reinforced through simulation. As the program of studies develops, more of the instruction becomes situated in actual clinical practice.

Components of the situated learning model include cognitive apprenticeship, coaching, multiple practice, and reflection.[17] Each of these components are used extensively in the transitional phase of the anesthesia program. Classroom content is reinforced in the simulation laboratory where students participate in a cognitive apprenticeship with the faculty as concepts are explored in a "real world" atmosphere. In the situated learning environment, the role of the teacher as a lecturer is replaced with the teacher as coach. During initial experiences, faculty are very active in instruction, first by modeling, then by providing direction as needed at critical points and eventually fading into the background as the student becomes more self-sufficient. The variable sensitivity of the simulator enables the teacher to coach through different techniques. Not only can the teacher coach by fading in and out of a procedure during difficult phases, but also the teacher can vary the difficulty of each simulation exercise. Initial simulations can be planned using robust patients requiring simple interventions and the difficulty of the exercise increased as the student progresses. As desired, the support of a teacher can be completely eliminated by allowing the students to use the simulator without supervision. To the student this may represent the final step in the progression from assisted to independent practice; however, as the student continues with the training, additional instruction may be necessary when challenging or stressful situations are encountered.[18] The instructor should be prepared to promote student-initiated corrective behaviors or to review aspects of an earlier lesson.

Two components of situated learning are introduced early in the educational program and are used as recurring themes. The first theme is collaboration. In the initial phases of the educational program, students work together to develop appropriate technical skills. As the program progresses, students work together and with faculty to solve complex problems. One of the important goals in developing these cooperative partnerships is to encourage students to learn to work together toward a common goal. It is intended that this cooperative approach be incorporated in patient care situations with individuals working together as a team in order to optimize patient care.

The second recurring theme is reflection, as described by DA Schön (The Reflective Practitioner. New York, Basic Books, 1983). Problems in clinical practice are viewed as complex unique situations which include uncertainty and conflicting values. Appropriate solutions to problems require both specialized knowledge and judgement.[19] As part of the reflective process, students evaluate their own performance. Through simulation, clinical situations can be recreated, alternative management strategies tested, and decision making reviewed.

There are two advantages for using an simulated environment for situated learning. First of all, there is the opportunity to design an interaction containing the hallmarks of a rewarding experience including high degrees of interaction and feedback, specific goals, a continuous feeling of challenge, a sense of direct engagement with the activity, the availability of appropriate tools to aid in the solution, and an environment that does not destroy the subjectiveness of the experience.[20] Secondly, teaching moments can be optimized as both the student and instructor participate in a simulation sequence with a common sense of purpose as compared to the uncontrolled nature of the operating room where the student and faculty may have different educational objectives, teaching may compete with service, extraneous circumstances events may present themselves unexpectedly, or instructor intervention is required to prevent possible morbidity or mortality.

6. CONCLUSION

We have integrated simulation throughout a curriculum for the preparatory education of nurse anesthetists. The design of our program is conducive to the use of simulation to reinforce didactic content and encourage situated learning. In fact, because of the critical care experiences of our students, simulation has the potential to be a more effective instructional medium for nursing anesthesia than in other areas of educations.

REFERENCES

1. Abenstein JP, Warner MA: Anesthesia providers, patient outcomes, and costs. Anesth Analg 1996;82:1273–83
2. Fallacaro MD: A look at anesthesia workforce projections. AANA News Bull April 1996;50
3. Qualifications and capabilities of the Certified Registered Nurse Anesthetist. Park Ridge, IL, American Association of Nurse Anesthetists, 1992, p 3
4. Gunn IP: Health education costs, provider mix, and healthcare reform: a case in point-nurse anesthetists and anesthesiologists. AANA J 1996;64:48–52
5. Beutler JM: Other perspectives on anesthesia. Health Aff 1988;7(4):20
6. Education and Research Department. AANA study of underserved, small, and rural hospitals. Park Ridge, IL, American Association of Nurse Anesthetists, 1994
7. Standards for Accreditation. Park Ridge, IL, Council on Accreditation of Nurse Anesthesia Educational Programs, 1994
8. Education and Research Department. Questions and Answers About a Career in Nurse Anesthesia. Park Ridge, IL, American Association of Nurse Anesthetists, 1996
9. Blumenrich GA: The standard of care. AANA J 1992;60:529–531
10. Masters FL, Skidmore MV, Thibideaux, BL: U.S. Army/Texas Wesleyan University program in anesthesia nursing. AANA J 1991;59:480–1
11. Byrnes GT: Current and future perspectives regarding the framework for nurse anesthesia education: military education of nurse anesthetists and the case for centralized academic program with multiple clinical affiliates: U.S. Navy. AANA J 1991;59:490–1
12. Vygotsky LS: Mind in Society: The Development of Higher Psychological Processes. Cambridge, MA, Harvard University Press, 1978
13. Brown JS, Collins A, Duguid P: Situated cognition and the culture of learning. Educational Researcher 1989;18:32–42
14. Tripp SD: Theories, traditions, and situated learning, Situated Learning Perspectives. Edited by McLellan H. Englewood Cliffs, NJ, Educational Technology Publications, 1996, pp 155–166.
15. Wertsch JV, Minick N, Arns F: Creation of context in joint problem-solving, Everyday Cognition. Edited by Rogoff B, Lave J. Cambridge, MA: Harvard University Press, 1984, pp 151–171
16. Ausabel DP: Education Psychology: A Cognitive View. New York, Holt, Rinehart, & Winston, 1968
17. McLellan H: Situated learning: Multiple perspectives, Situated Learning Perspectives. Edited by McLellan H. Englewood Cliffs, NJ, Educational Technology Publications, 1996, pp 5–17
18. Tharp RG, Gallimore R: Rousing Minds to Life. Cambridge, England, Cambridge University Press, 1988
19. Harris IB: New expectations for professional competence, Educating Professionals: Responding to New Expectations for Competence and Accountability. Edited by Curry L, Wergin JF. San Francisco, Jossey-Bass, 1993, pp 26–27
20. Norman D: Things That Make Us Smart. Reading, MA, Addison-Wesley, 1993

6

WHAT CAN YOU DO WITH A SIMULATOR?

Quality Assurance

Vimal Chopra

Department of Anesthesiology
University Hospital Leiden
P.O. Box 9600
2300RC, Leiden, The Netherlands

1. QUALITY, QUALITY ASSURANCE, AND QUALITY IMPROVEMENT

Quality is defined differently by different individuals.[1] The Concise Oxford Dictionary[2] defines it as "the degree of excellence of a thing". For medical care, quality can be defined as "that kind of care which is expected to maximize an inclusive measure of patient welfare, after one has taken account of the balance of expected gains and losses that attend the process of care in all its parts."[3]

Quality assurance (QA) refers to activities which monitor the quality of a service and may include methods to improve it.[1] QA has three components: structure, process and outcome (Fig. 1). *Structure* represents all components of the organization or department. These include administration, the place of work (environment, physical plant, operating room), personnel who carry out the work (anesthesiologists, residents, nurse anesthetists), and the equipment used (anesthesia machine, monitors). *Process* refers to measures which describe the operation of the system. These measures define what is done (tasks) and how it is done (methods). *Outcome* represents the effects of the care. From patient's point of view, outcome is defined by mortality and morbidity. From anesthesiologist's point of view, it includes unexpected alterations in planned care, such as unanticipated admission to intensive care or events requiring corrective actions.

Quality improvement is the effort to improve the level of performance of a process. It involves measuring the level of current performance, finding ways to improve that performance and implementing new and better methods.[1]

2. SIMULATORS AND ANESTHESIA

The practice of anesthesia involves routine activities which nonetheless have the potential of developing into critical incidents. Anesthesia training requires about 4–5 years

Simulators in Anesthesiology Education, edited by Henson and Lee.
Plenum Press, New York, 1998.

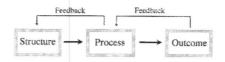

Figure 1. Components of a quality assurance program.

during which the trainee learns to give anesthesia under supervision. Many life threatening anesthesia emergencies have an incidence of one in 10,000 or less. It is possible that an anesthesiologist can complete his or her training without being exposed to these situations. Some anesthetic emergencies are so rare that most anesthesiologists may not even come across them during their professional career. An often quoted example of such an emergency is malignant hyperthermia. Anesthesiologists are expected to maintain their competence in managing these complications by reading textbooks, journals or attending appropriate lectures or refresher courses. This is passive learning. However, as in most other walks of life, anesthesiologists best retain their knowledge by active rather than passive learning. Even the routine skills used during anesthesia require constant vigilance and ability to handle problems that are immediately life threatening. In this respect anesthesia has much in common with other industries, such as aviation and the nuclear power industry. In these industries, simulators and training devices have been used for many years to maintain the efficiency and proficiency of their operators. These techniques are particularly highly developed in aviation where advanced technology provides realistic simulator systems for training and certification of airline pilots. The present generation of aircraft simulators are so realistic that pilots, who have been certified to fly one specific type of aircraft, are trained and certified to fly another type of aircraft (for example, a Boeing 747-400) entirely on the simulator.

The principal objective of simulators is to provide the highest transfer of skills from the training device to the operation systems.[4] Simulators improve the efficiency of training by allowing repetition of routine activities.[5] They also offer the possibility to practice rare emergencies. For example, in a flight simulator, a pilot can safely handle critical incidents like an engine fire or failed landing gear. While a pilot may log hundreds of hours of flight time without experiencing these situations, they can be created at will in a simulator.

Simulators are also used for evaluation. Certification and re-certification of pilots are partly accomplished by simulated sessions. Simulators can also be used to screen candidates for a particular task. Psychological testing has been carried out in simulators. Observations of the responses of personnel in a simulated environment can also lead to changes in the design of the original system. Ergonomics, the study of man-machine interfaces, has been influenced in this way.

3. ANESTHESIA SIMULATORS

Some authors differentiate a true simulator from a training device.[6,7] A simulator mimics the environment and phenomena as they appear in the real world. So, an anesthesia simulator should provide a learning experience that has a look and feel of a real operating room and real patient. Simulators are good for training and expert practice but are not necessarily good for the systematic learning of new skills and knowledge.

A training device, on the other hand, is more focused on teaching specific skills. It systematically presents to the trainee only the necessary training stimuli, feedbacks, reinforcements, remediations and practice opportunities, depending upon the trainee's learning level and style. Real world cues and phenomena are used only to a degree necessary to enhance the learning process.

Manikins for training intubation and resuscitation techniques and fiberoptic laryngo-bronchoscopy can be called training devices. Berge et al[8] describe a training device for detecting equipment failure in anesthetic machines. Their system consists of a modified anesthesia machine which allows 20 different preset technical faults to be activated from a control unit.

Educational programs that use only a computer screen display to present anesthesia information are training devices. Here the trainee learns by interacting with the computer program; the so-called computer assisted instruction or computer aided learning. Many such programs that mathematically simulate the uptake and distribution of inhalation agents (for example, Gas Man, ANSIM, Gas Uptake Simulation) and pharmacokinetics of intravenous agents (for example, TIVA-Sim) have been developed and evaluated.[9–14]

Gaba[15] classifies anesthesia simulators into three categories, namely realistic simulators or hands-on simulators; computer screen-only simulators or microsimulators and virtual reality simulators. A comprehensive classification of anesthesia simulators and training devices is shown in Table 1.

3.1. Computer Screen-Only Anesthesia Simulators

In the computer screen-only simulators or microsimulators, the entire anesthesia work environment is represented on a computer screen. These simulators are less expensive, more widely available, more flexible and can be more easily adapted to a specific user's needs. However, they lack the ability to simulate reality and certain important aspects of anesthesia practice, for example, the human-machine interactions and interactions between personnel. Two such currently available simulators are Anesthesia Simulator Consultant and BODY simulation.

The *Anesthesia Simulator Consultant* (ASC) was developed at the University of Washington, Seattle.[6,16–18] It operates on a personal computer and comprehensively simulates general anesthetics by creating graphical representations of patient, operating room equipment and displays on a computer screen. It evaluates an anesthesiologist's skills in management of routine and critical events. Mathematical models of physiology and pharmacology are used to predict the simulated patient's responses to anesthetic and other drugs and to pathological changes. The program includes a number of critical incidents which can be preselected by the user or at random by the computer. The expert system, which can be activated at any time during the case, gives critique, advice and instruction to the user. This group has also developed other interactive simulation programs such as Rhythm & Pulse, which is a cardiac life support training program and Critical Care Simulator, which repro-

Table 1. Classification of anesthesia simulators and training devices (reproduced with permission[40])

Anesthesia training devices
- Computer assisted instruction programs, e.g. Gas Man, TIVA-Sim
- Part-task trainers, e.g. intubation and resuscitation manikins

Anesthesia simulators
- Computer screen-only simulators e.g. ASC, BODY
- Full-Scale or realistic simulators, e.g. CAE, HPS, LAS, Sophus
- Virtual reality simulators

duces patient care in the intensive care unit and emergency department. These simulation programs are commercially available (AneSoft Corporation, Issaqquah, Washington).

Smith and Starko[19] described another PC-based anesthesia simulator called the *BODY simulation*. BODY simulates a patient; an anesthesia workstation with a ventilator and an anesthesia machine; parts of the operating room and even some operating room personnel on the computer screen. The program, which was originally called SLEEPER, is based on complex computer models which represent physiological functions and pharmacological actions and interactions. There are five screens which represent the patient, the anesthesia machine, the monitors, the drug trolley and the anesthetic record chart. This simulator makes it possible to study the mechanisms behind the clinical events in great detail, and teaches physiology and pharmacology in interesting ways.

3.2. Full-Scale Anesthesia Simulators

Full-scale or realistic anesthesia simulators recreate the anesthesia work environment in which the mock patient and equipment look, feel and behave as they do in real life. The anesthesiologist can give anesthesia under conditions which are as real as currently possible. These simulators however, are expensive to purchase and maintain. The commercially available full scale anesthesia simulators cost anywhere between $150,000 and $200,000. In addition, these simulators need adequate space and manpower to use them effectively. This incurs additional running costs.

3.2.1. Commercially Available Full-Scale Anesthesia Simulators. The *CAE Patient Simulator* (CAE Electronics Inc., Binghamton, New York) is a modified and improved version of the Comprehensive Anesthesia Simulation Environment (CASE) system. This simulator contains complete models of cardiovascular, pulmonary, fluid, acid-base and thermal physiology. The software is based on that of ASC. There is a full body computer controlled manikin with a computer system. A drug recognition system and a remote control interface have recently been added. CASE system, which was originally developed by a team at the Stanford University in California, was extensively used to study the responses and the decision making process of anesthesiologists while handling critical incidents and crisis situations during anesthesia.[20–25] The simulator was set up in an operating room and was used to conduct a new type of training course in anesthesia, called the Anesthesia Crisis Resource Management (ACRM) course.[26–29] Since the idea of "crew coordination" is the key element in this training, operation room nurses and surgeons play important roles (as themselves) during the course's simulation sessions. The CAE Patient Simulator is currently being used in several anesthesia training centers.[30]

The *Human Patient Simulator* (Medical Education Technologies, Inc., Sarasota, Florida) is a commercial modification of the Gainesville Anesthesia Simulator. This simulator, which is developed at the University of Florida in Gainesville, also replicates the clinical anesthesia environment.[7,31,32] It comprises a patient manikin that exhibits important clinical signs (for example, pulses, lung and heart sounds, twitch responses, spontaneous breathing), an anesthesia gas machine and mechanical ventilator, standard monitoring equipment, data acquisition and control hardware and microcomputers running physiological models and scenario-control software. The simulator is a model driven, script controlled system. Mathematical models of physiology and pharmacology form the basis of the software.[33,34] This simulator is currently being used in various centers in the United States and Japan for training and teaching basic skills and advanced techniques to anesthesiologists, residents and students.[35–38]

3.2.2. Non Commercial Full-Scale Anesthesia Simulators. The *Leiden Anesthesia Simulator* (LAS), developed at the University Hospital Leiden in the Netherlands, makes use of a standard anesthesia machine and monitoring devices.[39,40] It can be used with most commercially available anesthesia equipment and monitors, which are connected to the simulated patient just as they are to a real patient. A modified commercially available resuscitation manikin attached to an electro-mechanical lung model represents the simulated patient. The lung allows both spontaneous and mechanical ventilation. Physiological signals (ECG, arterial, pulmonary arterial and central venous pressure waveforms) generated by a signal generator and controlled by a personal computer provide input to the monitors. There are facilities for simulating non-invasive blood pressure measurement and pulse oximetry. The software responsible for the computer control of the simulated parameters is implemented on a 486-version personal computer and is based on a series of physiological and pharmacological models, which control interactions between the cardiovascular and the respiratory parameters.

LAS is currently installed in an actual operating room and is an integral part of the recently established anesthesia training center in Leiden, the *Anesthesiology Skills Lab* (Fig. 2). This facility also includes a fully dedicated briefing and debriefing room located within the operating room complex. The Skills Lab is being used for training and continuing education of anesthesiologists, anesthesia residents and anesthesia nurses throughout the Netherlands. New residents in Leiden are taught the basic principles of anesthesia on the simulator. The simulator is also used for evaluating the performance of residents. Anesthesia personnel are made familiar with new anesthesia equipment on the simulator before its clinical use. Evaluations of the ergonomic design and performance of new anesthesia equipment have been carried out on LAS.[41]

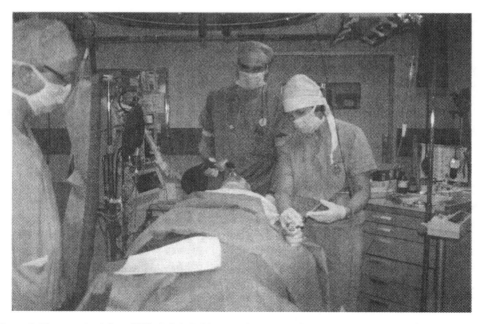

Figure 2. The Anesthesiology Skills Lab in Leiden. The full-scale Leiden Anesthesia Simulator is installed in an actual operating room.

The *Sophus Anesthesia Simulator*, developed by a team from Herlev Hospital, Roskilde University and Risø National Laboratory in Denmark, also uses real anesthesia equipment to recreate the operating room environment.[42] This full-scale simulator consists of a manikin, a PC and an interface module. The software used in this simulator consists of comprehensive cardiovascular and multi compartmental pharmacologic models. Software generated physiological signals are fed to real anesthesia monitors. This simulator has been in use for more than three years for training anesthesiologists in dealing with critical incidents during anesthesia. Evaluations conducted by the Sophus group have shown the need for improvement in anesthesiologists' knowledge of algorithms and procedural skills.[43–45]

The Sophus group has recently started a series of courses called "Rational Anesthesia".[46] These courses are based on the Crew Resource Management course conducted in commercial and military aviation and are analogous to the ACRM course developed at the Stanford University. The participants undergo a training program in which they receive instructions in diagnostic and treatment strategies about selected critical incidents. The importance of good coordination, leadership and communication while handling critical incidents during anesthesia is emphasized. Until now, more than 400 anesthesiologists and anesthesia residents in Denmark have undergone these courses.

The *Wilhelm Tell Simulator* was installed in 1994 at the University Hospital in Basel in Switzerland (H.G. Shaefer and D. Betzendörfer, personal communication, 1995). This is a total operating room simulator which consists of an anesthesia simulator and a surgical training device. The anesthesia simulator is a replica of the Sophus simulator. The surgical training device, which was developed at the Kantonsspital in Basel, offers training for laparoscopic surgery. The Wilhelm Tell simulator is installed in a dedicated location which includes a simulated operating room and a conference room.

This simulator is currently being used to conduct the Team Oriented Medical Simulation (TOMS) training sessions. This approach allows integrated training of the whole operating room team. Each team (anesthetic and surgical) has meaningful tasks to perform and the interactions among the participants are realistic. Like in most simulator centers, the TOMS training includes extensive briefing before and debriefing after the simulator session.

The *PatSim Simulator* was developed in Stavanger in Norway by a team of bioengineers with the purpose of training anesthesia and intensive care personnel (A. Rettedal, personal communication, 1995). Like other full-scale simulators, PatSim consists of a PC controlled manikin which can be placed either on an operating table or an intensive care bed. It can be ventilated. Laryngospasm, changes in lung compliance and airway resistance, pneumothorax, lung sounds, pulmonary secretions, gastric regurgitation and diuresis are electromechanically simulated. To date this simulator has been used in a limited way to train anesthesia and intensive care nurses in Norway. Efforts are now underway to use it for training anesthesiologists and anesthesia residents.

A relatively simple full-scale anesthesia simulator was described by Byrne et al.[47] The *Anesthesia Computer Controlled Emergency Situation Simulator* (ACCESS) system is designed to simulate anesthetic emergencies with the objective of improving the training of junior doctors. The simulator is based on standard anesthesia equipment, with a microprocessor providing an image of commonly used instruments. The presented problems are designed to test the skills of the trainees.

3.3. Virtual Reality Simulators

Virtual reality is a more imaginative way of providing a human-computer interface as compared with the familiar keyboard, mouse and screen system.[48] The medical application of virtual reality is currently limited to minimally invasive surgery, laparoscopy and endoscopy. One Nottingham-based group has recently reported having developed a virtual reality simulation system for anesthesia.[49] The technology is expensive at present and requires considerable time and resources to tailor it to specific needs. Moreover, bulky computers and headsets make the system difficult to use. However, with the current pace of development one can expect to get an affordable and manageable virtual reality anesthesia simulator within the next few years.

4. ROLE OF ANESTHESIA SIMULATORS IN QUALITY ASSURANCE

Where do currently available anesthesia simulators fit into the quality assurance model? Their obvious use as education and training tools to maintain the efficiency and proficiency of anesthesia personnel makes them fit into the first component of QA program, namely the structure. These could also be used as means to evaluate the performance of personnel and equipment and for research.

4.1. Teaching and Training

In anesthesia, as in other branches of medicine, the clinical skills are learned "on the job", i.e. by diagnosing and treating patients with problems under supervision. This is a productive and economical way of training new practitioners. Since simulator training is not expected to shorten the training period of anesthesia personnel, it will not reduce training costs.[5] On the other hand, the use of simulators brings in additional costs. Therefore, in order to make effective use of this training method, one must define the objectives clearly. What should be taught? Who should be taught and trained and how often? What organisational changes are needed in order to conduct this type of training? Teaching new residents the techniques of endotracheal intubation using anesthesia simulators, for example, is not cost effective. A simple intubation manikin is sufficient for this purpose.

The major purpose of anesthesia simulators is to rehearse management of both frequently occurring and rare events during anesthesia.[50–52] The computer screen-only simulators allow training on the concepts and procedures in handling uncomplicated and complicated cases. Full-scale simulators are ideal for teaching anesthesia residents and experienced anesthesiologists the concepts of human-machine interactions and the complications of working in a complex environment. Full-scale anesthesia simulators in many centers throughout the world are currently being used to conduct specialized courses and training sessions based on the concepts of Crew Resource Management courses developed by commercial and military aviation. Evaluations in Leiden have shown that simulator-based training and practice lead to a significant improvement in handling malignant hyperthermia.[53] During these evaluations, all participants had been given simulator training but only half were given training in the management of MH. When tested in the simulator four months later, those who were trained in the management of MH performed significantly better than those who had not undergone this training. The advantages of simulators as training tools are summarized in table 2.

The simulation environment also provides a vehicle for practice before the first experience. Simulator centers at Gainesville and Leiden have developed curricula for teaching basics of clinical anesthesia to new residents.[35,39] The Gainesville group have shown that simulation can accelerate learning of basic anesthesia skills by new residents.[36]

Table 2. Advantages of simulators in anesthesia
(reproduced with permission[40])

- No risk to patient
- Scenarios involving uncommon but serious problems can be presented
- Same scenario can be presented to many trainees
- Scenarios can be repeated
- Errors can be allowed without any risk to the patient
- Simulation can be stopped for teaching, and can be restarted

In anesthesia, when a new apparatus, drug or technique is introduced, the anesthesiologist more often than not learns to use this "on the job". Anesthesia simulators could be used to train anesthesiologists with new anesthetic equipment or techniques in a simulated environment, before their first clinical use in the operating room on a patient. This not only will increase the confidence of the users of the equipment and new techniques but will also contribute to the safety of patients.

4.2. Continuing Education, Evaluation, and Recertification

In comparison with professional pilots, anesthesiologists are not compelled to undergo any form of retraining and it is perfectly possible for someone to qualify in his early thirties and to continue a career in anesthesia until retirement age without ever attending a postgraduate course or other form of postgraduate education. This is far from an ideal situation. Clearly sound training, retraining and education of anesthesiologists will help reduce the incidence of mishaps. Perhaps formal retraining, proficiency checks and recertification should be made mandatory, for example once every year. This could be partially accomplished in a suitable anesthesia simulator. Routine in-training examinations, assessment of residents with questionable competence and periodic reexamination of practitioners can be conducted on simulators.

Use of anesthesia simulators to evaluate the performance of residents and experienced anesthesiologists is difficult at present.[15] Even the most realistic simulators cannot represent the patient perfectly. Moreover, a simulated crisis could be managed perfectly satisfactorily in many different ways. Only a trained expert anesthesiologist will be able to judge the actions of anther anesthesiologists properly. There are at present no well accepted standards for performance evaluation using anesthesia simulators. Assessment methods, based on the proficiency checks used for evaluating the performance of airlines pilots, are being evaluated by the Stanford group.[54] In spite of these difficulties some centers are using simulators to assess the performance of their residents.[39]

4.3. Research

As a research tool, a simulator can be used to study the responses of anesthesia personnel to critical incidents, to evaluate the utility of different displays or alarm modalities, the effects of artifacts or false alarms on problem solving performance and effect of fatigue and other stresses on anesthesiologists' performance. The Stanford team have used their simulator extensively to study the responses of anesthesiologists to simulated critical incidents, the effect of experience on the performance of anesthesiologists in managing such incidents and the role of fixation error in managing simulated critical incidents.[21–25] Other research areas that can be addressed using anesthesia simulators include the cognitive science of dynamic decision making, human-machine interactions, teamwork and the possible role of intelligent decision support systems in anesthesia and intensive care.[15]

4.4. Evaluation of Equipment

Anesthesia simulators can be used to evaluate the ergonomics and performance of new anesthetic equipment. Dynamic testing of equipment using a simulated anesthetic crisis provides the manufacturer with useful information about the performance and the ergonomic design of the equipment.[41] Such information helps them to suitably modify the equipment design. This can be particularly useful during the development phase of the equipment, and helps in improving the user friendliness of the equipment. The use of simulator in this situation can result in considerable savings in development costs.

5. FUTURE DEVELOPMENTS

Until recently only few training centers had access to an anesthesia simulator. Now there are more than 20 centers throughout the world that have an anesthesia simulator installed. Many more are considering acquiring one and their number is expected to rise rapidly. Anesthesia simulators will undoubtedly become more advanced as they incorporate future technological developments. Sophisticated physiological and pharmacological models have been developed and implemented on computers to control the simulated parameters more effectively. In spite of all these, as compared with the aircraft simulators, it is extremely difficult, if not impossible to simulate all types of patient variations perfectly. Even healthy patients show considerable biological variability.

The manikins used in full-scale anesthesia simulators are the least realistic in simulating reality. Skin and temperature changes, eye signs and patient movements are not simulated realistically. A more realistic manikin capable of simulating some of the patient responses will add considerably to the realism of the simulators. Manikins used in commercial and non-commercial full-scale simulators are constantly being improved. Virtual reality is another exciting development. One can certainly expect to hear more about it in the years to come.

Simulation in anesthesia is developing rapidly. However, much fundamental research is still needed to achieve the tremendous potential of simulators in our specialty.

REFERENCES

1. Eagle CJ, Davies JM: Current models of "quality": an introduction for anesthetists (review). Can J Anesth 1993; 40:851–62
2. Allen RE (ed): *The Concise Oxford Dictionary of Current English*. Oxford: Oxford University Press 1990
3. Donabedian A: Promoting quality through evaluating the process of patient care. Med Care 1968; 6:181–202
4. Blaiwes AS, Puig JA, Regan JJ: Transfer of training and the measurement of training effectiveness. Human Factors 1973; 15:523–33
5. Schwid HA, O'Donnell D: Simulators and anesthesia training. In: Eichhorn JH (ed). *Problems in Anesthesia: Improving Anesthesia Outcome*, Vol 5(2). Philadelphia: J.B. Lippincott Company, 1991; 319–28
6. Andrews DH: Relationships among simulators, training devices, and learning: A behavioral view. Educational Technology 1988; 28:48–54
7. Good ML, Gravenstein JS: Anesthesia simulators and training devices. International Anesthesiology Clinics 1989; 27:161–6

8. Berge JA, Gramstad L, Jensen Ø: A training simulator for detecting equipment failure in the anesthetic machine. European Journal of Anesthesiology, 1993; 10:19–24

9. Heffernan PB, Gibbs LM, McKinnon AE: Teaching the uptake and distribution of halothane: a computer simulation program. Anesthesia 1982; 37:9–17

10. Heffernan PB, Gibbs JM, McKinnon AE: Evaluation of a computer simulation program for teaching halothane uptake and distribution. Anesthesia 1982; 37:43–6

11. Philip JH, Lema MJ, Raemer DB, Crocker D: Is computer simulation as effective as lecture for teaching residents anesthetic uptake and distribution? Anesthesiology 1985; 63:A503

12. Philip JH: Gas Man - an example of goal oriented computer-assisted teaching which results in learning. International Journal of Clinical Monitoring and Computing 1986; 3:165–73

13. Paskin S, Raemer DB, Garfield JM, Philip JH: Is computer simulation of anesthetic uptake and distribution an effective teaching tool for anesthesia residents? Journal of Clinical Monitoring 1985; 1:87–8

14. Tanner GE, Angers DG, Van Ess DM, Ward CA: ANSIM: An anesthesia simulator for the IBM PC. Computer Methods and Programs in Biomedicine 1986; 23:237–42

15. Gaba DM: Human work environment and simulators. In Miller RD (ed). *Anesthesia.* New York: Churchill Livingstone, 1994; 2635–79

16. Schwid HA: A flight simulator for general anesthesia training. Computers and Biomedical Research 1987: 20:64–75

17. Schwid HA, O'Donnell D: The anesthesia simulator-recorder: a device to train and evaluate anesthesiologists' responses to critical incidents. Anesthesiology 1990; 72:191–97

18. Schwid HA, O'Donnell D: *Anesthesia Simulator Consultant (User's Reference Manual).* Bellevue: University of Washington and Anesoft Corporation, 1990

19. Smith NT, Starko K: PC-based anesthesia simulators. Society for Computing and Technology in anesthesia News 1995; 8:8–9

20. Gaba DM, DeAnda A: A comprehensive anesthesia simulation environment: re-creating the operating room for research and training. Anesthesiology 1988; 69:387–4

21. Gaba DM, DeAnda A: The responses of anesthesia trainees to simulated critical incidents. Anesthesia and Analgesia 1989; 68:444–51

22. DeAnda A, Gaba DM: Unplanned incidents during comprehensive anesthesia simulation. Anesthesia and Analgesia 1990; 71:77–82

23. DeAnda A, Gaba DM: Role of experience in the responses to simulated critical incidents. Anesthesia and Analgesia 1991; 72:308–15

24. Botney R, Gaba DM, Howard SK, Jump B: The role of fixation error in preventing the detection and correction of a simulated volatile anesthetic overdose. Anesthesiology 1993; 79:A1115

25. Botney R, Gaba DM, Howard SK: Anesthesiologist performance during a simulated loss of pipeline oxygen. Anesthesiology 1993; 79:A1118

26. Gaba DM: Dynamic decision making in anesthesiology: cognitive models and training approaches. In: Evans DA, Patel VL (eds). *Advanced Models of Cognition for Medical Training and Practice.* Berlin: Springer Verlag GmbH, 1992; 123–47

27. Howard SK, Gaba DM, Fish KJ, Yang G, Sarnquist FH: Anesthesia crisis recourse management training: teaching anesthesiologists to handle critical incidents. Aviation, Space & Environmental medicine 1992; 63:763–70

28. Holzman RS, Cooper JB, Small S, Gaba DM: Participant responses to realistic simulation training in Anesthesia Crisis Resource Management (ACRM). Anesthesiology 1993; 79:A1112

29. Gaba DM, Fish KJ, Howard SK: *Crisis Management in Anesthesiology.* New York: Churchill Livingstone, 1994; 31–47

30. Gaba DM: Simulator training in anesthesia growing rapidly: patient simulators used for resident, CME courses. Anesthesia Patient Safety Foundation Newsletter 1995; 10:34–6

31. Good ML, Lampotang S, Gibby GL, Gravenstein JS: Critical events simulation for training in anesthesiology. Journal of Clinical Monitoring 1988; 4:140

32. Good ML, Gravenstein JS: Training for safety in an anesthesia simulator. Seminars in Anesthesia 1993; 12:235–50

33. Heffels JJM: *A Patient Simulator for Anesthesia Training: A Mechanical Lung Model and a Physiological Software Model.* Eindhoven: EUT Report 90-E-235, ISBN 90–6144–235–4, 1990

34. van Meurs, WL, Beneken JEW, Good ML, Lampotang S, Carovano Jr RG, Gravenstein JS: Physiologic model for an anesthesia simulator. Anesthesiology 1993; 79:A1114

35. Good ML, Gravenstein JS, Mahla ME, White SE, Banner MJ, Carovano RG, Lampotang S: Anesthesia simulation for learning basic anesthesia skills. Journal of Clinical Monitoring 1992; 8:187–8

36. Good ML, Gravenstein JS, Mahla ME, White SE, Banner MJ, Carovano RG, Lampotang S: Can simulation accelerate the learning of basic anesthesia skills by beginning anesthesia residents? Anesthesiology 1992; 77:A1133
37. Öhrn MAK, van Meurs W, Good ML: Laboratory classes: replacing animals with a patient simulator. Anesthesiology 1995; 83:A1028
38. Euliano T, Good ML: Simulator training in anesthesia growing rapidly. Anesthesia Patient Safety Foundation Newsletter 1996; 11:7–9
39. Chopra V, Engbers FHM, Geerts MJ, Filet WR, Bovill JG, Spierdijk J: Leiden anesthesia simulator. British Journal of Anesthesia 1994; 73:287–92
40. Chopra V: anesthesia simulators. In: Aitkenhead AR (ed). *Baillière's Clinical Anesthesiology: Safety and Risk Management in Anesthesia* 1996; 10(2):297–315
41. Chopra V, Bovill JG: Evaluation of a patient monitor using an anesthesia simulator. Anesthesiology 1995; 83:A1064
42. Jensen PF, Ørding H, Lindekær AL, The Sophus Group: The anesthesia simulator Sophus. Abstracts of the 9th European Congress of Anesthesiology 1994:A169
43. Lindekær AL, Jensen PF, The Sophus Group: Anesthesiologists management of unexpected anaphylactic shock during anesthesia in a full scale anesthesia simulator-Sophus. Abstracts of the 9th European Congress of Anesthesiology 1994:A28
44. Lindekær AL, Jensen PF, The Sophus Group: European anesthesiologists managing unexpected ventricular fibrillation in a full scale anesthesia simulator Sophus. Anesthesiology 1994; 81:A1275
45. Gardi Ti, Jensen PF, Ørding H, The Sophus Group: How do anesthesiologists treat MH in a full-scale anesthesia simulator? British Journal of Anesthesia 1995; 74:A73
46. Christensen UJ, Laub M, The Sophus Group: The Sophus anesthesia simulator. British Journal of Anesthesia 1995; 74:A72
47. Byrne AJ, Hilton PJ, Lunn JN: Basic simulations for anesthetists: a pilot study of the ACCESS system. Anesthesia 1994; 49:376–81
48. Burt DER: Virtual reality in anesthesia. British Journal of Anesthesia 1995; 75:472–80
49. Lloyd C: Anesthetists learn to operate in virtual reality. Sunday Times, London: 16 April 1995.
50. Gravenstein JS: Training devices and simulators (editorial). Anesthesiology 1988; 69:295–7
51. Gaba DM: Improving anesthesiologists' performance by simulating reality (editorial). Anesthesiology 1992; 76:491–4
52. Chopra V, Bovill, JG: Improving anesthesia safety. In: Taylor TH, Major E (eds). *Hazards and Complications of Anesthesia,* 2nd edition. Edinburgh: Churchill Livingstone, 1993; 13–25
53. Chopra V, Gesink BJ, de Jong J, Bovill JG, Spierdijk J, Brand R: Does training on an anesthesia simulator lead to improvement in performance? British Journal of Anesthesia 1994; 73:293–7
54. Gaba DM, Botney R, Howard SK, Fish KJ, Flanagan B: Interrater reliability of performance assessment tools for the management of simulated anesthetic crises. Anesthesiology 1994; 81:A1277

7

TEAM ORIENTATED MEDICAL SIMULATION

Stephan C. U. Marsch[*]

Department of Anesthesia
University of Basel
Kantonsspital, 4031 Basel, Switzerland

1. INTRODUCTION

Team orientated medical simulation (TOMS) stands for high-fidelity full scale simulation of a complete operating room including all personnel usually involved in the patients' care. This novel approach to training in the medical field was first performed at the University of Basel in Switzerland in December 1994 under the leadership of Hans-Gerhard Schäfer (figure 1). After the death of Hans-Gerhard in July 1995 his work has been carried on by a team of investigators from both the anesthetic and surgical departments of the University of Basel as well as coworkers from outside the institution. To the best of our knowledge, the simulator situated in the University of Basel is still the only one used to train complete operating room teams.

TOMS is part of scientific project at the Department of Anesthesia of the University of Basel investigating the impact of human factors in the operating room. Besides TOMS this project includes systematic observations in the operating room, surveys on attitudes of operating room personnel, a quality assurance program, and an anonymous critical incidence reporting system (CIRS) on the internet.

2. BACKGROUND

The impact of human factors and communication on the performance of operating room teams remains to be determined. However, every practitioner is well aware that the presence of skilful professionals per se is no guarantee against the occurrence of critical incidences or disasters. Examples of these complications include mix up of patients or operations. There is good evidence that in high-risk environments critical incidents are associated with poor communication and interface problems.

---

[*] For the TOMS team: Dieter Betzendörfer, Ewald Duitmann, Christoph Harms, Robert Helmreich, Irene Klöti, Thomas Kocher, Stephan Marsch, Olaf Schellscheidt, Daniel Scheidegger, Christoph Schori, Bryan Sexton, Urs Zenklusen

Simulators in Anesthesiology Education, edited by Henson and Lee.
Plenum Press, New York, 1998.

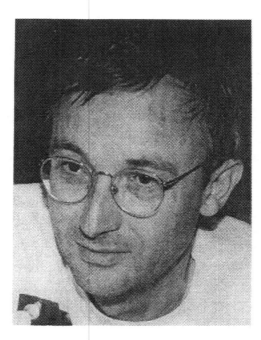

Figure 1. Hans-Gerhard Schaefer (1951–1995), the "father" of TOMS.

Even in comparison with other high-risk technological domains (aviation, nuclear power station) an operating room has to be considered a highly complex environment. The technological reliability and sophistication is such that the occurrence of disasters due to failure of equipment are extremely rare. Instead, patient's condition and human errors are the main cause for critical incidents.

Many different health-care professionals are involved in the perioperative management of any single patient. In addition to differences in personality, operating room personnel differs in background (academic, non-academic), training, and status. Moreover, though the physical presence of several individuals suggests an operation to be a team endeavour, one has to recognise that different subgroups or subteams (anesthesia, surgery, nursing) are involved, each team having its own culture. Thus, failure in communication may occur at the interface between teams as well as within any single team.

The common goal of all individuals and groups in the operating room is the safety of their patients. In addition, the increasing economic constraints make the efficient use of resources in the operative medicine mandatory. Both patients' safety and efficiency depend on interactions between individuals and teams. In other high-risk environment the implementation of simulator training rather than introduction of new technology was found to improve safety. In the medical field, simulation has been successfully employed to practice skills while avoiding potential damage to patients. The rationale for team orientated medical simulation (i.e. full operating room simulation) is to train individuals and teams in communication skills required to perform their task.

Team training cannot replace in-depth professional education. Instead technical proficency of all personnel involved in the patients' care is a prerequisite for team training to be efficient and successful. Thus, TOMS is not competing with other groups using simulators for improving skills of anesthetits and surgeons. However, our approach of a human factor training for highly specialised and qualified personnel is novel in the medical field and recognises the need for education that goes beyond individual professional compentence.

3. THE SIMULATOR

The simulator is situated on the hospital campus remote from the building of the operating rooms. The simulator is essentially a room that has been transformed in a operating theatre and allows high-fidelity simulation of surgery and anesthesia (figure 2). Special care was taken to ensure that all equipment is identical to that used in the real operating room. The 'patient' (nicknamed Wilhelm Tell) consists of a commercially available resuscitation mannequin and an abdominal laparoscopic simulator. The mannequin is equipped with an intravenous line and may be intubated and mechanically ventilated. Monitoring include ECG, invasive and non-invasive blood pressure, pulseoximetry, and capnography. Laparoscopic surgery is performed on porcine abdominal organs (preparation including gut, kidneys and aorta) obtained from the slaughterhouse. Prior to the simulation the organs are cannulated and connected to a perfusion pump so that bleeding can be simulated using red dye.

Haemodynamic variables and oxygen saturation are controlled by software specifically designed for this purpose. In order to obtain a realistic capnogram carbon dioxide is fed into the low-pressure circuit of the ventilator.

Inevitably a mannequin is not a real patient and there are a number of things a mannequin cannot do (e.g. sweat, cough, move on incision). Moreover, the software cannot detect kind and amount of drug injected into the mannequin. These problems are solved by the presence of a member of the TOMS team (nicknamed 'interface') in the operating

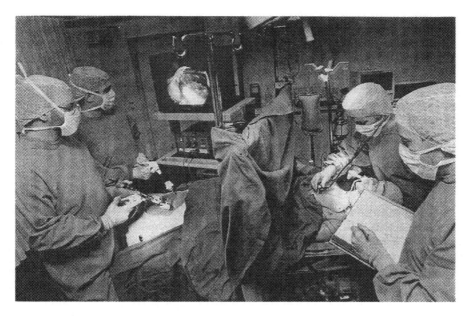

Figure 2. Partial view of the full-scale operating room simulator at the University of Basel. Laparoscopic surgery is performed during general anesthesia.

room. The interface communicates with his colleagues outside the operating room and passes on, on request, information to the participants that is otherwise not available due to technical shortcomings of the mannequin.

4. THE SIMULATION

The philosophy of our project is that all personnel normally involved in the care of a patient in the operating rooms of our institution take part in a simulation. Participants include orderly, anesthetic nurse, anesthetic resident, anesthetic consultant, scrub nurse, surgical resident, and surgical consultant resulting in a number of 7 persons involved in each simulation. In addition, at least three memebers from the TOMS group are required to run a simulation.

Simulations are scheduled on the official daily operating program. Since during simulations participants are not available to perform clinical work, the departments of surgery and anesthesia agreed on closing one regular operating room on the simulation day. Prior to the simulation both surgical and anesthesia resident receive charts of their 'patient'. The charts include patient's history, clinical examination, laboratory results, and radiographs. Together with their consultants the residents review the charts and formulate a plan for surgery and anesthetic management respectively.

The simulation consists of three parts: briefing, simulation, and debriefing. The purpose of the briefing is to inform participants on the aims of human factors training. Confidentiality and the intention to train and learn rather than to evaluate are especially emphasised.

After a technical briefing the simulation starts and laparoscopic surgery is performed during general anesthesia. It is our philosophy not to test the limits of skills and knowledge of any individual participant. Instead we select scenarios that require communication and interactions within and between teams, e.g. pneumothorax or bleeding. To facilitate the simulation to be a positive experience we have so far ensured that the 'patient' will not die or suffer serious damage. This policy might be changed once all personnel of our institution is used to simulations.

The simulation session is videotaped. Besides the visual information the tape contains recordings of wireless microphones attached to every participant. During the debriefing the participants will share their experiences of the simulation and sequences of the videotape are viewed and discussed. In addition, implications of teambehaviour experienced during simulation for the 'real' operating room are discussed.

5. ACHIEVEMENTS OF TOMS

Due to the manpower necessary to carry out simulations, so far only one simulation day per month with two simulation sessions each was possible. However, all simulation scheduled could be performed even in times of shortage of personnel. Thus, a major achievment of the TOMS group is the acceptance of the project within their institution.

Participant evaluation of TOMS indicate strong acceptance of the training with no difference between the different subgroups involved. Moreover, the realism of the scenario received favourable ratings indicating that we achieved a good standard of simulation. A more extensive discussion of these topics may be found in our abstract 'participant evaluation of team orientated medical simulation' printed in this book.

Discussions with many participants revealed that the TOMS program resulted in an awareness of communication and team issues. Moreover, the mere possibility to watch oneself on videotape during the debriefing was found to be an important experience.

Observations performed in the operating room and the survey on attitudes of the operating room personnel provided us with a baseline of communication and attitudes prior to the start of the simulator training. A more extensive overview on observational data may be found in our abstract "jumpseating in the operating room" printed in this book.

6. FUTURE PROJECTS

Regular observations and surveys are planned in order to assess the impact of TOMS on attitudes of personnel and team behaviour in the operating room.

One has to recognise that interactions between teams and communication in an operating room are inherently different from aviation and probably much more complex. Though the use of methodology validated in aviation (observation, simulation) proved very useful in avoiding to start a process from a zero base, it is mandatory to modify procedures in order to meet the specific needs of operating room personnel.

8

WORKSHOP ON EDUCATIONAL ASPECTS

Educational Objectives and Building Scenarios

W. Bosseau Murray[1,2] and Lindsey C. Henson[1,2]

[1]Simulation Development and Cognitive Science Laboratory
Pennsylvania State University College of Medicine
Milton S. Hershey Medical Center
Hershey, Pennsylvania
[2]Department of Anesthesiology
University of Rochester School of Medicine
Rochester, New York

1. INTRODUCTION

The purpose of this workshop was to define the process of creating learning objectives and using them to build scenarios on the simulator. Human patient simulators are best used to teach the more complex levels of cognitive knowledge—those defined by Bloom[1] as "analysis," "synthesis," and "evaluation." Using simulators in medical education, whether for medical students, anesthesia residents, anesthesiologists, or others, is extremely labor-intensive on the part of the faculty. Therefore, simulators should be used to teach levels of knowledge which cannot be taught as effectively by more traditional and less costly methods, such as lectures, readings, problem sets, or small group discussions. In order to make the most of a simulator, the learning objectives should be defined before designing the simulator scenario, and the first question to ask is: Is the simulator the best way to achieve these learning objectives? The learning objectives should drive the use of the simulator and the scenario, rather than the reverse. The simulator is a tool which is only as good as the time spent by the educational objective writer. However, it is a very good tool when used effectively to teach the appropriate level of knowledge.

The following topics were covered during this workshop:

Steps in designing scenarios for the simulator

> Define the goal/purpose
> Define the audience
> Define the time available

Simulators in Anesthesiology Education, edited by Henson and Lee.
Plenum Press, New York, 1998.

Define the learning objectives
   Objectives based upon the Levels of Knowledge
      Bloom's Taxonomy of Cognitive Knowledge
      Practical session: small group discussions

Matching objectives with the correct teaching tool

Building scenarios

2. STEPS IN DESIGNING SCENARIOS FOR THE SIMULATOR

2.1. Define the Goal/Purpose

The first step is to define the broad goal or purpose of the teaching session. This can be phrased in non-technical and non-educational terms (avoiding educational jargon), which allows all teachers to reach consensus in the briefest possible time. For example, the PBL (Problem Based Learning) organizers at Pennsylvania State College of Medicine wished to obtain some "practical" experience for their second-year medical students on the simulator. Their request stated simply "Do something on the pulmonary artery catheter (PAC)" for the basic course. These same organizers requested another PBL session as an advanced subject later in the year, which was stated as "Patient in right ventricular failure vs. left ventricular failure, using the PAC." The Department of Anesthesiology at the same institution required training for residents on the management of the patient with a difficult intubation (an expert subject for residents). The request was "Sign off on the ASA (American Society of Anesthesiologists) Difficult Airway Algorithm."

Each of these requests states a broad goal or objective. The simulator faculty can then define more specific objectives which can be used to design the scenario. For instance, for the "Do something on the PAC" goal, the specific objectives might be:

1. Recognize the normal pressure wave forms and patterns for the SVC, RA, RV, and PA.
2. Know how the PAC is used to determine cardiac output and peripheral vascular resistance.
3. Use the PAC to diagnose and treat shock.

For the "Sign off on the ASA Algorithm" goal, the specific objective might be:

Recognize and respond appropriately and in a timely fashion to the "Cannot Intubate, Can Ventilate" and "Cannot Intubate, Cannot Ventilate" situations. In order to be "signed off," the resident's response must follow the ASA Algorithm and the patient must survive.

2.2. Define the Audience

The second step is to garner as much information as possible about the audience. Determine the following:

- What is the level of existing knowledge of the trainee/learner ?
  - Is it high or low?
  - Is it known or unknown?
- Are these active or passive learners?
- What is the group size?
  - Is the group size controllable or not controllable?

The existing level of knowledge of the audience will determine what type of learning objectives can be achieved and whether a preliminary session to bring all learners "up to speed" is needed. The learning style of the audience will often determine not only the type of simulator session (small group for active learners, large group demonstration for passive learners) but also whether it makes sense to use the simulator at all. One advantage of the simulator may be to convert passive to active learners; at the University of Rochester we find that, by inviting participation in a non-threatening way, the faculty can often engage the more passive medical students in a group of 5–6 in hands-on activities and decision-making.

Group size is one of the major determinants of successful or unsuccessful simulator sessions; whenever possible the organizers should strive for the smallest possible group size. Group size determines how much hands-on experience can be given to each participant. A group size of two allows each participant to do once and observe once, allowing reinforcement of principles. A group size of three, with each participant observing twice, is also good for beginners. Larger group sizes, with multiple repetitions of the same scenario, may become tedious but can be managed by using different and/or increasingly complex scenarios. However, not all learners will have the opportunity to actually repeat the hands-on part of each scenario. If the group size cannot be controlled, the session must be planned to use the simulator best for the predetermined number of students.

While the simulator can be used to teach large groups, the objectives need to be quite different. The simulator becomes a demonstration, rather than a hands-on training experience. We have used the simulator to demonstrate principles of compliance and resistance of the lungs/chest wall with first-year medical students at the University of Rochester; the simulator was set-up in a large classroom with video cameras trained on the monitors and a "lecture/demonstration" format was used. Students were asked to explain changes in peak inspiratory pressure, plateau pressures, and volumes delivered by the ventilator based on their understanding of compliance and resistance; these topics had already been taught at the "factual knowledge" level by other instructors. The session was very successful, but it used the simulator for teaching at the lower levels of knowledge (Bloom's "comprehension" and "application", see below). To address "analysis," "synthesis," and "evaluation," a different format with smaller groups of students would be needed. Such sessions have been used at the Penn State College of Medicine for new residents during their "First Three Days" in the residency program[2] as well as for Second Year Problem Based Learning (PBL) medical students.

To obtain a suitable group size, we often have to arrange multiple stations with content related to the specific simulator session. For instance, a station with anatomy of the airway may complement a simulator session on the difficult airway. The small group size is one reason simulator training is so expensive in terms of teacher time. The perceived value of the simulator session offsets this expense.

2.3. Define the Time Available

The third step is to decide how much time will be set aside for the training session. Ask yourself:

Does the time allow

- a brief introduction to simulator?
- an in-depth study of diagnostic methodology?
- repetitive psycho-motor practices and/or drills?

Grandiose ideas often have to be tailored to fit the minimal time that is realistically available.

2.4. Define the Learning Objectives

The fourth step is to define specific learning objectives, which requires determining what types of knowledge should be presented to the participants. One classification of types of knowledge that is useful in designing learning objectives for the simulator is Bloom's Taxonomy, which breaks cognitive knowledge into 6 progressively deeper/higher levels of knowledge[1]. These levels of knowledge are intended to be hierarchical. In addition to defining each level of knowledge, it is valuable to consider how the students can demonstrate that they have attained this knowledge (since this guides us in how to "test" our students). Bloom's Taxonomy can be distilled as follows:

- FACTUAL KNOWLEDGE: Recall of specifics, of ways of dealing with specifics, or of the major patterns by which ideas are organized; demonstrated by bringing information to mind without changing it.
- COMPREHENSION: Knowing what is communicated and being able to use it; demonstrated by paraphrasing, summarizing, or extrapolating from information.
- APPLICATION: Using abstractions in concrete situations; demonstrated by remembering generalizations or principles and bringing them to bear on a new problem.
- ANALYSIS: Breaking down material into constituent parts and recognizing relationships between them; demonstrated by distinguishing facts from hypotheses, checking the consistency of hypotheses against a set of data, or detecting causal relationships.
- SYNTHESIS: Drawing on information from many sources and putting them together into a structure not clearly there before; demonstrated by producing a plan to test an hypothesis or by formulating an appropriate hypothesis to explain data.
- EVALUATION: Making judgments about the value of ideas based on either internal consistency and logical accuracy or in reference to external criteria. This level of knowledge is the most difficult to demonstrate; in medical decision-making, it often entails evaluating the response of the patient to treatment derived from analysis and synthesis and may require the learner to cycle back through these two processes in order to come to the correct diagnosis.

To demonstrate the use of Bloom's Taxonomy, consider the example of these levels of knowledge applied to the game of golf.

- FACTUAL KNOWLEDGE: I know the rules of golf.
- COMPREHENSION: A rough is an area with deep grass outside where the ball is supposed to be during play.
- APPLICATION: I am faced with a short hole. I know that a nine iron is designed to hit the ball a short distance. I will use a nine iron for this hole.
- ANALYSIS: The less shots I hit the better my score. To decrease the number of shots I have to choose the right clubs.
- SYNTHESIS: I have never tried this shot before, but I think the distance is 130 yd and I can usually hit the ball 130 yd with a nine iron so I will use a nine iron for this shot.
- EVALUATION: I missed that last shot with the nine iron because the wind was in my face and the shot was uphill, so I will try it next time with an eight iron.

If we go back to the example of the learning objectives for the "Do something with the PAC" scenario, we can further refine these objectives and also start to plan which learning objectives are better taught with the simulator and which can be addressed in a less labor-intensive format. First, break down the objectives according to Bloom's Taxonomy. The original objectives were:

1. Recognize the normal pressure wave forms and patterns for the SVC, RA, RV, and PA.
2. Know how the PAC is used to determine cardiac output and peripheral vascular resistance.
3. Use the PAC to diagnose and treat shock.

Using Bloom's Taxonomy, these objectives become:

- FACTUAL KNOWLEDGE: Define shock and list typical abnormalities, including changes in systemic and central hemodynamics. Recognize the normal pressure tracings for the SVC, RA, RV, and PA. List normal values for these pressures. List factors measured by the PAC which determine cardiac output and peripheral vascular resistance.
- COMPREHENSION: Explain the pathophysiology of 3 types of shock (hypovolemic, cardiogenic, distributive/septic).
- APPLICATION: Based on your knowledge of the pathophysiology of the 3 types of shock, design and explain appropriate therapy. Predict the direction of abnormalities of central hemodynamics with the 3 different types of shock.
- ANALYSIS: Examine and analyze the history, signs, symptoms and vital signs (including tracings and calculations from the PAC) in a specific patient to predict the type of shock and the extent of abnormalities.
- SYNTHESIS: Develop a treatment plan for this patient. Based on the previous analysis, plan appropriate therapy (combining information garnered above.)
- EVALUATION: Evaluate the effects of therapy (IV fluids, inotropic drugs, etc.) on cardiovascular parameters to determine if the diagnosis and treatment plan are correct and effective. Which therapy should be tried first (is the best), fluids or inotropic agents?

We believe the simulator experience to be of increasing value for the more complex levels of knowledge (perhaps application, certainly analysis, synthesis and evaluation). Thus, for the "Do something with the PAC" scenario, students can cover the objectives for the first three levels of knowledge in the classroom in a large group or in small-group discussions. The simulator, on the other hand, can be used to present them with a specific patient with a specific type of shock and allow them to analyze that patient's disease process, develop a treatment plan, evaluate the effects of their treatment, and cycle back through analysis, synthesis, and evaluation as needed to successfully correct the abnormalities[3].

During the workshop, participants were divided into small groups (5–6 per group) and given the following instructions on a hand-out, which included a description of Bloom's Taxonomy as outlined above, including the definitions of each level of knowledge.

Write one or two learning objectives for each level of knowledge, with the overall goal of teaching the differential diagnosis of tachycardia. The actual cause of the tachycardia will be anaphylaxis/anaphylactoid reaction.

Each group was asked to write one or two learning objectives for each of the levels of knowledge in the taxonomy. The only other guideline given was that the objectives should be based on "do" words and that they should try to avoid questions on pure factual knowledge, since the simulator is best used for the higher levels of knowledge. The small groups were given the following information about steps 1–3 as outlined above:

Step 1. Define the goal/purpose

- Management of tachycardia

  - Not reflex administration of a β blocker for the tachycardia
  - Not treatment of a single number (heart rate)
  - Think about the cause of the tachycardia—establish a differential diagnosis including anaphylaxis/anaphylactoid reaction

Step 2: Define the audience

- Second year anesthesia residents

Step 3. Define the time available

- One hour for a group of 2 residents working together

The following learning objectives for this overall goal were developed by the small groups during the workshop. Participants noted that the "do" words are more difficult to write and use as objectives, because we are not used to thinking and teaching this way.

- FACTUAL KNOWLEDGE: Define normal heart rate (HR). Define normal heart rate for a specific patient. Define tachycardia. List a differential diagnosis of tachycardia.
- COMPREHENSION: Recognize that increased heart rate can be either abnormal or normal or even a compensation to the decreased blood pressure of induction of anesthesia. Describe signs from the cardiovascular system that indicate increased HR is abnormal. Understand normal control of HR and effects of various perturbations. Explain the pathophysiology of tachycardia.
- APPLICATION: Given a male with a femur fracture and a pulse rate of 110 beats per minute—what does this mean? Explain or recognize other signs and symptoms which suggest anaphylaxis.
- ANALYSIS: Derive options—are the signs and symptoms from Applications present or not? Track down the cause. Figure out why, *i.e.*, differential diagnosis. Analyze the history, signs, symptoms and vital signs in a specific patient to determine the cause of increased HR.
- SYNTHESIS: Use diagnostic criteria and/or pattern recognition to develop a treatment plan.
- EVALUATION: Evaluate the response to therapy—fluids ⇒ no effect ⇒ other signs and symptoms ⇒ back to analysis and synthesis and re-evaluate. Evaluate and compare different forms of therapy.

3. MATCHING OBJECTIVES WITH THE TEACHING TOOL

Once the objectives have been defined, the following important question should be asked: *Is the simulator the best method to attain/teach/demonstrate/learn each objective?* If the objectives include words such as "define," "list," "recognize," or "explain," we can teach this with a White Board or a Flip Chart in a group session (saving lots of time and teacher energy); a simulator is not needed for such basic knowledge transfer. On the other hand, if the objectives include higher/deeper levels of cognition, such as "manage," "diagnose and treat," "adjust treatment plans according to response to therapy," "do the right things first," "don't waste time," or "check equipment as a cause," we do need a good simulator. The human patient simulator is not the best way to teach pharmacokinetics; a dedicated computer program which models levels of drug in various compartments would be more effective. It is not the best way to teach arrhythmias or detection of myocardial ischemia by ST depression on the EKG because the fidelity of the simulators are not yet good enough. It is an excellent way to teach students to recognize and treat complex problems that present with common signs, such as tension pneumothorax or cardiac tamponade. It is invaluable for teaching uncommon problems such as malignant hyperthermia[4]. Another excellent use is teaching trouble-shooting with equipment problems.

If you have decided that the simulator is the right tool for the learning objectives, determine if the students need to have an introductory talk on the knowledge base or the teaching tools (*i.e.*, the simulator and monitors). Students will get much more out of a simulator session addressing the learning objectives in the analysis, synthesis, and evaluation levels if they have had a prior discussion or review of the objectives in the factual knowledge, comprehension, and application levels. For complex algorithms, such as ACLS (Advanced Cardiac Life Support) or the ASA Difficult Airway Algorithm, the students need to have an overview as well as knowing the details of each path before being able to apply their knowledge. It can be confusing to work through a branch of the algorithm without an understanding of the "big picture."

4. BUILDING SCENARIOS

Once the objectives have been clearly defined and you have decided to use the simulator, develop a story line to accomplish these objectives. The story line should be believable, whether it is a typical case (easier for both the instructor and the student) or an atypical and therefore more difficult case[4,5]. The story line should not be too complex, or the student will get bogged down in side issues and never address the objectives. For example, in the anaphylaxis scenario, tachycardia developing immediately after induction and intubation or immediately after administration of an antibiotic will be less confusing than tachycardia developing after several other events. Students should be given any background information about the patient or situation that they will need. For anesthesiology residents, this can take the form of a written preoperative evaluation or a "sign out" (hand over) from the anesthetist previously taking care of the patient. For the anaphylaxis scenario, this information may simply be "This is a healthy 22 y/o male patient who has sustained a femur fracture. All other evaluation is negative and the cervical spine has been cleared."

For the anaphylaxis scenario, the objectives developed in the small groups included recognizing not only an abnormal heart rate but other signs and symptoms of anaphylaxis, which include some that can be reproduced with the simulator (hypotension, increased airway pressures) and some that cannot (hives). The scenario should be constructed such that the students are be able to figure out what is going on without the latter type of visual information. Other issues to consider are whether to let the patient die if the student completely misses the diagnosis; administration of a ß-blocker in a patient with severe anaphylaxis may result in this outcome. Faculty may decide that this event is a good way to reinforce another of the learning objectives ("don't respond to one number, look at the whole patient"). The scenario can then be re-started to explore and "evaluate" other approaches to the problem. Ideally, the scenario should end when the student has achieved the learning objectives. For anaphylaxis, this means that the students have given epinephrine *and* know why (either because they figured out the diagnosis and knew how to treat, or because they tried epinephrine and figured out the diagnosis based on the patient's response).

Commercially available human patient simulators have many scenarios "built-in" (preprogrammed) which can often be used directly or with only slight modifications. Almost all anesthetic and vasoactive drugs are also preprogrammed. Whether we are using a preprogrammed scenario or one we have written ourselves, we run through it and try a variety of possible student reactions to see what will happen. There are still some surprises; for the anaphylaxis scenario, the student may confuse ACLS doses of epinephrine (milligrams) with those needed to treat anaphylaxis (micrograms.) Recently, the third-year medical students at the University of Rochester decided to treat an overdose of fentanyl, which resulted in apnea, with an entire ampoule of naloxone. The patient started to breathe again, but we had to quickly re-institute "pain" by giving epinephrine.

We usually try to make the overall simulator experience positive, even if it means "replaying" the scenario several times until the student succeeds. We do not believe in using the simulator as a "pass or fail" testing device. We prefer to present the simulator a "friend" which can help the trainee through multiple scenarios until successful treatment has been achieved.

REFERENCES

1. Bloom BS, Engelhart MD, Furst EJ, Hill WH, Krathwohl DR: Taxonomy of Educational Objectives. Handbook 1: Cognitive Domain. New York: David McKay Company, 1956.
2. Murray WB, Foster PA, Schneider AJL, Robbins R: The new residents' first 3 days: Measuring the efficacy of an introduction to clinical anesthesia with perceived self-efficacy scales. Anesthesiology 81: A1238, 1994 (Abstract).
3. Allen GC, Glenn JD, Murray WB, Riley J: Enhancing problem based learning using a human patient simulator. Presented at the Seventh Ottawa International Conference on Medical Education and Assessment, Maastricht, The Netherlands, June 25–28, 1996.
4. Gaba DM, Fish KJ, Howard SK: Crisis Management in Anesthesiology. Churchill Livingstone, New York:, 1994
5. Schneider AJL, Murray WB, Mentzer SC, Miranda F, Vaduva S: "Helper" - A critical events prompter for unexpected emergencies. J Clin Monit 1995;11(6):358–364

MODEL DRIVEN SIMULATORS FROM THE CLINICAL INSTRUCTOR'S PERSPECTIVE

Current Status and Evolving Concepts

Willem L. van Meurs and Tammy Y. Euliano

Department of Anesthesiology
University of Florida College of Medicine
Gainesville, Florida 32610

1. INTRODUCTION

The clinical instructor is facing several challenges when designing and teaching a full-scale simulator based course. As an educator, he or she has to define learning objectives, select or program scenarios that simulate a case that helps meet these objectives, and sometimes define a simulated patient that is more suited to meet a particular objective than the ones already provided by colleagues or by the simulator manufacturer. Knowing the strengths and limitations of these relatively new teaching tools is part of the challenge. Adding strength as well as challenge is the fact that in many educational simulations of human physiology and pharmacology, mathematical models have taken over the role of "simulation engine" from pre-selected ("scripted") vital signs. One advantage of such models is that they can take into account gradual variations of multiple management variables. Another advantage is that they can be made to reflect interactions between physiological subsystems, such as the ventilation and the circulation. A potential shortcoming of using mathematical models in educational simulations is complexity.

A first, general observation is that the mathematical models reflect the (natural) complexity of physiologic and pharmacologic phenomena. While familiarity with these phenomena is part of the background of the simulator instructor, this knowledge alone is not sufficient for interaction with the simulator models. Therefore, our purpose is to guide simulator instructors in facing this interaction, whereby we will use our dual experience as simulator developers and instructors. This experience was gained on the Medical Education Technologies, Inc./University of Florida Human Patient Simulator (METI/UF HPS). The concepts discussed in this paper are general in nature, and will apply to other full-scale simulators as well.

After a brief overview of modeling concepts, and of models in a full scale simulator, we will discuss different levels of instructor involvement. The use of pre-programmed sce-

Simulators in Anesthesiology Education, edited by Henson and Lee.
Plenum Press, New York, 1998.

65

narios (provided by colleagues, or by the simulator manufacturer) requires relatively little interaction with the simulator mathematical models. Programming of the physiology of a particular patient, necessary to meet an educational objective, is an exercise that requires more in-depth interaction with the models. In section 4.3 we will elaborate on an example: the programming of a specific patient physiology. We will conclude this chapter with a section of evolving concepts.

2. OVERVIEW OF MODELING CONCEPTS: VARIABLES, PARAMETERS, AND ESTIMATION

In engineering disciplines, it is common to make the following distinction between two types of entities, (adapted from Sévély[1]):

- *variables* are entities that change over time, and
- *parameters* are entities that are stable over time.

Variables can be further divided into (Fig.1):

- *independent variables or inputs:*

  - *control inputs* are entities that may be modified (voluntarily) to make a system evolve. Examples of control inputs in anesthetic management are: administered drugs and fluid volumes, inspiratory gas fractions, and ventilator settings.
  - *disturbances* are inputs that affect a system independent of the controller's will. Examples of disturbances are: blood loss, sudden changes in metabolism as during malignant hyperthermia, and endogenous catecholamine release during laryngoscopy.

- *dependent variables*:

  - *state variables,* intuitively speaking, contain the "memory" of a system. State variables and subsequent inputs together completely determine the evolution of a system. Examples of state variables in anesthetic management are: compartment blood volumes, blood gas contents, drug concentrations, and alveolar gas concentrations. The state variables determine if the patient is in induction or emergence, the patient's volume status, etc. As will be clear from the examples, state variables are not necessarily directly measurable or alterable entities.
  - *outputs* are functions of inputs and state variables: blood pressure, heart rate, and end-tidal gas values are clinical examples of outputs.

Parameters are the constants in a mathematical description of a system relating input, current state, and output. Examples of parameters in anesthetic management are:

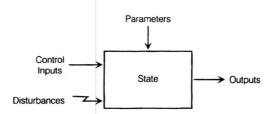

Figure 1. Diagram of multiple variables.

body weight, tissue volumes, and anesthetic gas solubility coefficients (for a fixed body temperature).

In the medical field, the distinction between parameter and variable is not always as clear as in the engineering sciences. For example, systemic vascular resistance (SVR) is considered a parameter when it is used to describe the relationship between cardiac output and mean arterial pressure. When describing the effect of the baroreflex or the effect of a vasoconstrictor, SVR becomes a time-varying entity, and therefore a variable. In the simulator models we only consider the baseline SVR a parameter. Sometimes we use the term "independent parameter" if this parameter can be reset before or during a simulation run (this maintains the practical distinction with, for example, the constantly varying blood pressure).

Using this terminology, in model driven simulators, the *user interface* and scripted *scenarios* are used to set disturbances, to generate or override control inputs, or to set independent parameters. *Programming a scenario* consists of establishing the right sequence and magnitude of these changes. *Defining a patient* consists of 1) establishing a target set of vital signs (outputs), 2) finding a set of parameters and a set of initial state variables, so that the right outputs result in a (semi-)static situation, and 3) verifying that the outputs react in an appropriate way to dynamically changing inputs. Steps 3) and 4) are a *Parameter estimation* procedure, as illustrated in Fig. 2.

Parameter estimation is often an iterative process; based on a prediction error, a model parameter adjustment is made and the model prediction is compared to real system data (ideally for a representative range of inputs). A new, hopefully smaller, prediction error results, and a next parameter adjustment is made. In engineering problems parameter estimation is often accomplished by a computational procedure, minimizing some criterion on the prediction error. For the more complex patient-ventilator system a formal "parameter adjustment algorithm" is not always feasible. The adjustments in this context are carried out by the clinical educator, and vary from adjustments based on literature data about parameter changes to educated guesses about the changes in the underlying physiology. We will elaborate on examples of parameter estimations for a human patient simulator in section 4.

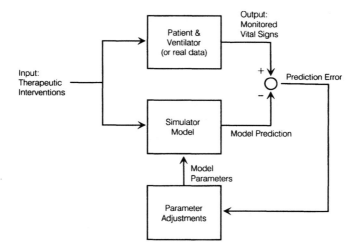

Figure 2. A parameter estimation procedure.

Several simulators have the capability to directly override the (dependent) monitored output signals. This may be practical to create a "steady-state", necessary to make a particular teaching point, but it reverts the simulator back to a script driven, static, and thus unphysiologic, system.

3. MODELS IN A FULL-SCALE SIMULATOR

Model driven full scale simulators elaborate on the multiple modeling approach pioneered by Beneken and Rideout2 and used in "screen-only" educational simulations.[3] One important aspect of full scale simulators is that, besides mathematical (software) models, they incorporate hybrid models (computer controlled mechanical models). Examples of the hybrid models in the METI/UF HPS are ventilation and gas exchange. Table 1 lists the main mathematical and hybrid models of the METI/UF HPS models and their interactions. Note that the inputs and outputs of these models are not listed in this table.

Designing a scenario or a patient usually requires interaction with only a subset of these models, but because of the multiple interactions, caution is required when setting parameters of a single model. For example, the interaction between ventilation and the circulation, through intrathoracic pressure, can have a significant effect on cardiac output. Describing each model in detail is beyond the scope of this paper. In section 3.3: defining patient (patho)physiology, we will refer to the cardiovascular model in more detail.

In the METI/UF HPS, the fast acting physiologic control mechanisms: baroreflex and the control of spontaneous breathing, are implemented in the following way: *control effectors*, such as heart rate or tidal volume, are modulated around a baseline reference, depending on the difference between *controlled variables*, such as mean arterial pressure and the partial pressure of CO_2 in the arterial blood (P_aCO_2), and their setpoint. In the initial phase of parameter estimation, it is often useful to eliminate this modulation. This is done by putting respective gains to zero. Then a desired "operating point" is established by adjusting input variables and the parameters that represent the baseline control effectors, so that target controlled variables result. For example, to obtain a certain combination of P_aCO_2 and breathing pattern, the baseline CO2 production, tidal volume, and respiratory rate, are adjusted. In a second stage, the controls are reactivated, and responses to dynamic changes in controlled variables (for example: ventilatory response to CO_2) are evaluated and adjusted.

4. INTERACTION WITH SIMULATOR MODELS

The main focus of this section will be on the definition of a patient by making model parameter adjustments. This topic will be covered in section 4.3. First, we will briefly describe two other levels of interaction with the simulator models.

4.1. Instruction Using Pre-Programmed Scenarios

The level of interaction with the simulator models for an instructor who uses preprogrammed scenarios is limited to verifying that the simulator responds to therapeutic interventions as expected. If it does not, then the possible causes are (diagnosis requiring an increasing level of knowledge of the simulator models): inappropriate timing and/or magnitude of scenario changes, inappropriate baseline patient definition (model parameters),

Table 1. Interactions between the mathematical and hybrid models of the METI/UF Human Patient Simulator (HPS). Planned, but not yet implemented interactions are indicated by brackets

FROM \ TO	Cardiovascular	Lung mechanics	Pulmonary gas exchange	Systemic uptake and distribution	Pharmacokinetics	Cardiovascular PC and PD	Respiratory PC and PD
Cardiovascular	—		Pulmonary blood flow	Blood volume and flow in tissue	[Cardiac output, blood volume]	Mean arterial pressure	
Lung mechanics	Intrathoracic pressure	—	Gas flow rates and volumes				[Lung stress receptors]
Pulmonary gas exchange		Net gas exchange	—	Alveolar partial pressures			
Systemic uptake and distribution	O_2 saturation of arterial blood		Central venous partial pressures	—		PO_2 in the brain	PO_2 in arterial blood, PCO_2 in the brain
Pharmacokinetics					—	Effector site drug concentrations	Effector site drug concentrations
Cardiovascular PC and PD	Heart rate, contractility, SVR, capacitance					—	
Respiratory PC and PD		Respiratory muscle pressure					—

PC = physiologic controls; PD = pharmacodynamics

and model limitations. Sometimes it is necessary to verify expectations by consulting the literature. In our minds, two factors can improve this verification (and adjustment) process: clear documentation, targeted at clinical instructors, and an expanded role of the simulator technician to include knowledge about the simulator models.

4.2. Programming Scenarios, Using Existing Patients

As stated in section 2, programming a scenario consists of establishing the right sequence and magnitude of disturbances, control inputs, and independent parameters. This requires a deeper knowledge of—and experience with—the responses of a simulator.

The same suggestions for facilitating this process as in the previous section can be made. For the commercially available simulators, we refer the instructors to the lists of parameters that can be modified through the user interface and with the patient editor.

4.3. Defining Patient (Patho)Physiology

The first step in defining a patient is to determine the goal and the extent of the simulation exercise that will be based on this patient. We distinguish three somewhat overlapping levels of patient definition: (1) the "complete" simulation of a well-described subpopulation, (2) a general simulation of a particular pathophysiologic state, and (3) a "single use" patient with certain conditions. These different types lead to variations on the "parameter estimation procedure" described in section 2. In this section we will focus on cardiovascular and respiratory physiology. Pharmacologic changes will be discussed in section 5.

4.3.1. Simulation of a Sub-Population. This level of patient definition is to describe a different "normal" physiology, for example a parturient or pediatric patient. There are several steps in the simulation of such a well-defined physiology:

1. Identify target vital signs: These may be found in the literature, or through clinical experience. Recall that vital signs data are *dependent* entities (section 2.1).
2. Determine physiologic alterations: The alterations must be described in the most basic parameters possible. For example, consider the determinants of blood pressure (Figure 3).
3. The most significant independent parameters include systemic and pulmonary vascular resistance (SVR/PVR), heart rate, contractility, venous capacity, and left ventricular compliance. Volume status (state variables) is also important in this case. Data for these parameters must be sought in the literature. In a second stage, changes in baroreflex sensitivity must be considered.
4. Incorporate into system: As mentioned before, deactivating the baroreflex, then manipulating the independent parameters and variables to achieve the target vital signs, is a practical means of developing a patient. Then, before reactivating the baroreflex, its pressure setpoint should be reset, such that it regulates the patient's mean arterial pressure appropriately.
5. Test: Once the parameters are programmed, run the patient and compare the resulting vital signs with the targets. It is also important to calculate resulting SVR and PVR as these may differ from the set baseline, once the control mechanisms are activated.
6. Return to step (2), seeking further physiologic alterations to resolve discrepancies between the simulated and target vital signs data. Since for most parame-

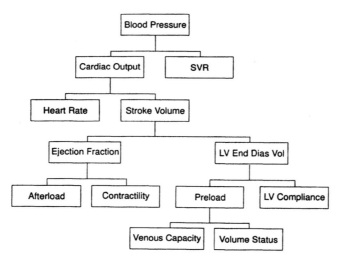

Figure 3. Physiologic determinants of blood pressure.

ters, literature review will result in a range of possible values, consider changing values within the range. Additionally, a search for additional parameters might also be necessary. Consider venous distensibility and aortic volume and distensibility. Inevitably there will be "holes" in the literature which will require best-guess estimation on the part of the programmer.

7. Test the dynamic responses of the simulated patient to perturbations (e.g. volume loss).

These steps should then be repeated for respiratory changes (keeping in mind that extreme ventilatory patterns may influence the cardiovascular system).

4.3.2. Simulation of a Patient with a Specific Pathology. This level of simulation is used to create patients with a particular condition, congestive heart failure, for example. These patients have a single pathologic condition with a certain severity. Literature data is available to define many of the alterations to independent parameters, but since clinically there is a wide range of "severity" and manifestations in individual patients, the programmer has much more lee-way in the patient definition. Again the first step is to identify target vital signs, these will vary with the learning objectives. Second is to determine physiologic alterations, using clinical knowledge and a pathophysiology textbook. These changes are incorporated into the system, tested, and then additional alterations are made as required. Unlike the detailed patient simulation, strict adherence to the literature is not essential, though physiologically reasonable changes are necessary (i.e., to simulate low blood pressure due to CHF, mostly contractility should be decreased, not SVR or volume status).

4.3.3. Simulation of a "Single Use" Patient. To teach specific learning objectives we often create a series of scenarios to be run on a single patient. The "single use" patient is designed in such a way that multiple etiologies for complications are reasonable (e.g. hypotension due to hemorrhage, pneumothorax, etc.). The patient is described in advance through a "case stem" which is then used to define the physiology. The patients' status and physiology is fully determined by the instructor's learning objectives. We will illustrate this concept through an example:

1. Define learning objectives: We wish to create a patient who will develop hypotension intraoperatively of various etiologies including hemorrhage, pericardial tamponade, tension pneumothorax and anaphylaxis.
2. Select physiologic alterations: The following is the case stem:
   A 52-year-old woman presents for a staging exploratory laparotomy for a probable ovarian malignancy. She has ascites, increasing shortness of breath and orthopnea with decreasing exercise tolerance. She has a 70 pack/year smoking history but is otherwise healthy. Vital signs include blood pressure 100/70 mmHg, pulse 120 bpm, respiratory rate 34 bpm, room air oxyhemoglobin saturation 93%. Chest X-ray reveals changes consistent with chronic lung disease, and echocardiogram shows a small effusion and ejection fraction of 45%.
   Physiologic alterations include:
   Cardiac: pericardial fluid, decreased ejection fraction, probable dehydration
   Pulmonary: rapid shallow breathing with normal breath sounds and increased shunt fraction
3. Select target vital signs: These are found in the case stem.
4. Incorporate alterations: Program the physiologic alterations into the simulator
5. Test: Run the simulation and compare the resulting vital signs with the targets
6. "Tweak": Make further alterations to the independent parameters until the desired targets are achieved. The selected alterations should be physiologically sound, that is, a true representation of the patient described.

5. EVOLVING CONCEPTS

In an interesting editorial in 1994, Dr. Asbury wrote: "As more drugs are developed and new anesthesia techniques are devised, simulators will need to be updated. Physically this will probably be easy to do, by software transfer. However, the software will probably need to be written by the company providing the simulator and provided at their prices. Potentially, simulator users could become locked-in to the manufacturer. No manufacturer wishing to preserve his market share will allow the local hospital physicist or a computer literate anaesthetist to update the simulator's programs; all key computer programs will probably be enciphered.[4]"

The existence of scenario and patient editors for both commercially available simulators partially belies this prediction. A major challenge lies in the education of simulator instructors about their teaching tool. Some of this educational need is met by the scenario and patient editors and associated documentation that are provided with both commercially available full-scale simulators. Experience with these new tools needs to be exchanged, and this conference certainly plays an important role in this context. The end goal is that the simulator instructor can fully focus on education, rather than how to interact with physiologic and pharmacologic models.

Addressing one of Dr. Asbury's concerns, a concept that is currently evolving is that of a pharmacology editor. There is considerable variability in pharmacologic responses between patients. Some of this variability can be predicted based on patient characteristics such as age, sex, weight, and height, or based on pathology. Some of the variability is less predictable[5]. A tool for adjusting the pharmacokinetics and pharmacodynamics of intravenous agents is currently under development at our institution.

For the long term, a few simulator development sites cannot provide all the mathematical or mechanical models that are required to meet diverse educational objectives for a variety of target groups. Examples of potential additions are models for intracranial pressure, or for a heart-lung machine for cardiopulmonary bypass. It is the opinion of the authors, that to be able to "tap" the enormous expertise at numerous simulator sites, an "open model architecture" should be provided. The table presented in this paper is an early attempt to clearly outline (sub)model boundaries, so that models can be replaced or added.

REFERENCES

1. Sévély Y.: Modélisation, simulation, contrôle, commande. Numéro spécial de BIOFUTUR "Biotechnologies et informatique," June, 1984.
2. Beneken, J.E.W., Rideout V.C.: The use of multiple models in cardiovascular system studies: Transport and perturbation methods, IEEE Trans. Biomed Engin, 1968;15:281–289.
3. Schwid H.A.: A flight simulator for general anesthesia training. Comput-Biomed Res 1987;20:64–75.
4. Asbury A.J.: Simulators for general anaesthesia, Editorial, Br J Anaesth, 1994;73:285–286.
5. Fiset P., Donati F., et al: Vecuronium is more potent in Montreal than in Paris, Can J Anaesth, 1991;38:717–721.

10

TECHNICAL WORKSHOP

Mathematical and Computer Models

David H. Stern

Department of Anesthesiology
University of Rochester School of Medicine
Rochester, New York

1. INTRODUCTION

Over the last few years, anesthesia simulation has advanced from purely screen-based simulations running on a desktop computer and consisting only of software, to the full-body simulator. The latter uses a computer system to control a life-size mannequin, which is equipped with lungs, a cardiovascular system, and other features which enhance realism and allow trainees to test motor skills as well as thought processes. The full-body simulator has electromechanical sensing and control devices. These allow software-dictated physiologic changes to be reflected in external monitoring devices (e.g. EKG, blood pressure) and in physically detectable characteristics (lung compliance, airway difficulty, muscle twitch, heart sounds). In addition, administered drugs, ventilation, and other external stimuli can be sensed by the system and reported back to the software.

There are two levels of computer programming involved with full-body simulators. The low-level code, which may be written in "C" or another computer language, dictates the physiologic and pharmacologic models which determine the basic behavior of the simulator. This is usually proprietary and cannot be changed by the user. Although at least one company is developing a drug editing module which will allow users to add or design new drugs, current simulators include a pre-programmed library of available drugs and associated pharmacokinetics and pharmacodynamics that cannot be changed by the user. In addition to the disk-based software that runs the simulator, peripheral interface modules can make use of "firmware" (programs stored permanently in a Read-Only Memory chip). These typically are used for storing digitized waveforms used as a library to construct EKG and pressure waveforms as well as heart and breath sounds.

This workshop was intended to demonstrate not how the low-level code is written, but rather how the user can use a built-in high-level programming language to create "scenarios". Scenarios are sequences of physiologic, pharmacologic, or other events which are used to create a particular disease process or complication. They can consist of a single initial set of physiologic specifications, such as a patient with ischemic heart disease or septic shock,

Simulators in Anesthesiology Education, edited by Henson and Lee.
Plenum Press, New York, 1998.

75

or a sequence of events that progresses over a set time period such as anaphylaxis, hemorrhage, ACLS algorithms, or malignant hyperthermia. When there is a series of events over time, the progression may be triggered manually by the operator, or automatically based on user-programmed transitions such as time, administration of a particular drug, or variations in ventilation or physiologic parameters. Events are often used in a fixed sequence, but may also be used in random fashion as the actions of the trainee dictate.

Two simulators were used for the demonstration: The "Human Patient Simulator" ("HPS") was formerly manufactured by Loral Corporation and is now sold by METI (Medical Education Technologies, Inc, a division of Lockheed Martin). The "Virtual Anesthesiology Training Simulator System" ("VATSS") is made by CAE Corporation. (Similar types of simulators are under development in Europe, but are not commercially available in the United States.) With both simulators, programmed scenarios can be designed "offline" on an isolated computer workstation without requiring the complete system of the instrumented mannequin and associated hardware.

The HPS is based on a PC-compatible computer using at minimum an Intel 80486 processor with a bus speed of 66 Mhz. The software will run with some limitations on a freestanding "PC" (IBM-compatible personal computer). This requires some minor changes to the HPS program configuration file to disable communication with the simulator's external devices via the serial interface or the analog-to-digital and digital-to-analog convertors. Communications between the main computer and the peripheral microcomputers and other devices is handled by software program modules called drivers.

The communications drivers enable the main PC to communicate with the peripheral microcontrollers and other devices that perform functions such as:

- operation of the mechanical lungs for spontaneous ventilation and simulation of lung compliance and other physical lung parameters
- analysis of inhaled gas concentrations and generation of appropriate physiologic exhaled gas mixtures which can then be detected by standard patient breathing circuit gas analyzers (CO_2, O_2, N_2O, Isoflurane)
- generation of heart and breath sounds via speakers inside the chest wall
- generation of ECG signals applied to external chest electrodes which are in turn attached via standard ECG clip leads to an external ECG patient monitor
- identification and dose measurement of a variety of intravenous drugs (currently by means of syringes labelled with bar-codes, and a sensitive scale to weigh the injected volume)
- generation of a pulse oximeter signal in an artifical finger that works with any standard oximeter sensor
- generation of pressure transducer signals for systemic arterial, pulmonary arterial, and right atrial pressure waveforms
- operation of an internal isoflurane syringe pump to deliver precise physiologic concentrations of isoflurane in the exhaled gas, corresponding with release of isoflurane from body tissues during emergence from anesthesia
- occlusion of the upper airway on command and control of left and right bronchial resistances

Simulators may use different means of driving external patient monitors. The HPS in most cases simulates actual physiologic signals, so that it can use standard "off the shelf" patient monitors from a variety of manufacturers. For example, a standard pulse oximeter sensor is placed on an artifical "finger" which detects the light from the oximeter sensor but then uses its own light source to produce the desired pulse rate and oxygen saturation.

Thus, the same oximeter sensor that would be placed on a real patient's finger can be used on the simulator. Likewise, the chest electrodes generate the same ECG signals that would be produced by an actual patient. The lungs exhale carbon dioxide which is sampled and measured by a standard airway gas analyzer.

The alternative is to use modified patient monitoring equipment that can accept electrical control signals, bypassing the actual patient sensor. This simplifies the design and enhances reliability because it eliminates mechanical factors, but has the disadvantage that specially modified, dedicated monitors must be used. The HPS and VATSS use both approaches to some extent. The HPS generates a pressure to mimic the oscillometric signal in the blood pressure cuff (though not the arm itself). For invasive pressures, however, electrical signals are generated so that the simulator interface replaces the pressure transducer and mimics the transducer's electrical output instead.

When the HPS software is run independently of the above peripheral hardware, the lack of any data for inhaled gas concentrations forces respiratory functions to remain fixed at baseline values (e.g. pH = 7.40, pCO_2 = 40). Although the automatic drug recognition system is absent, drugs are easily given (by bolus or infusion) using the keyboard or mouse. Obvious limitation are that heart and breath sounds can't be heard, chest compliance can't be felt, and EKG, pressure, and pulse oximeter waveforms cannot be detected. While the current software version does not yet allow real-time display of these waveforms, this is planned for a future version, and periodic digital values are currently recorded in a log file for later review.

The VATSS system is based on the SUN Microsystems workstation, which uses a high resolution graphical display. As noted above, the simulator's interface in many cases bypasses electromechanical transducers and sends its outputs directly to dedicated ports on the physiologic monitors. The current version lacks gas analysis (note: the new version of the VATSS will add respiratory functions and gas analysis); vaporizer and flowmeter settings are manually entered by the operator as they are changed. A new revision has recently added drug recognition by means of special electronic syringe interface modules, and injected volume is measured by a miniature flowmeter. Prior to that all drugs had to be entered manually by the operator. While the lack of active gas analysis and gas mixture generation to simulate real-time respiration limits realism and is not as physiologic a simulation, it does allow a more complete simulation to be run when the main computer is separated from the mannequin and other hardware. It is also possible to pause the CAE simulation, which is problematic in a real-time system using actual gases, since gases continue to flow and compositions continue to change. The CAE system displays physiologic waveforms directly on the simulator control screen, as well as the external patient monitor, which is a benefit when running a simulation without the full mannequin system. However, this feature is not necessary for designing most scenarios. In fact, regardless of which simulator is used, it will be necessary to fine tune the scenario on the full simulator because the physical interface can change its behavior.

Subsequent revisions of both simulators seem to be migrating toward a common design. The current HPS mannequin is similar to the VATSS, and rather than having the lungs built into the table below, the HPS mannequin will be connected to the other hardware by an umbilical cable in order to allow use of standard OR tables and beds. The scale-based drug recognition system generally works well but is sensitive to vibration and air bubbles, and if the trainee fails to turn the IV stopcock in the correct sequence, drugs may not be recognized. This will be replace by a new flowmeter-based drug recognition system similar to that used by CAE on the VATSS, and METI plans to add real-time physiologic waveform display to the control monitor in the future. CAE is adding real-time gas and respiratory functions.

However, both systems can currently be used without their peripheral hardware for purposes of user programming of scenarios. This allows scenarios to be developed "off-line" by many individuals on independent workstations without tying up the actual simulators.

Two demonstration workstations were set up in the meeting room.

2. SCENARIOS VS "ON-THE-FLY" PARAMETER CHANGES

Both simulators allow for changing individual cardiovascular, respiratory, and other parameters at any time during a simulation.

One approach to running a simulation is for the operator to start with a normal, healthy patient, and then to make individual changes to create problems. Examples might be:

- decreasing left ventricular contractility to simulate a patient with ischemic heart disease
- increasing bronchial resistance to simulate bronchospasm
- administering a small dose of epinephrine to simulate endogenous release of epinephrine in response to surgical stimulation in the presence of inadequate anesthesia

"On-the-fly" parameter changes allow great flexibility. It is possible to tailor the anesthetic course to present different complications to trainees depending on their responses, much like the conduct of an oral board exam. The operator can the change the scenario freely. On the other hand, this approach is highly labor-intensive. It is difficult for the simulator operator to work closely with the trainee, and a second faculty member is often required.

Scenario scripts allow either manual or automatic sequencing of events and physiologic changes. With a manually-advanced scenario, the operator simply presses a key to advance to the next event (for example, the start of an anaphylactic reaction, malignant hyperthermia, or sudden blood loss). Alternatively, the operator can skip randomly to any scripted event.

The next step in scenario sophistication is to add "transition statements", which are conditional tests that cause specific events to occur based on passage of time, plasma drug levels, or changes in physiologic parameters. A complex scenario can therefore run automatically with little or no intervention by the simulator operator, thereby freeing up a faculty member to work with the trainee. For example, an anaplylaxis scenario can automatically advance with time to progressively more severe bronchospasm and vasodilation, with automatic resolution when appropriate therapy is given.

3. WRITING SCENARIOS

As an example, we will contruct a scenario to model a morbidly obese patient for the HPS. Desired characteristics might be:

- Body weight of 140 kg with appropriate pharmacokinetics
- Decreased chest wall compliance with elevated inspiratory airway pressure
- Ventilation perfusion mismatch with rapid desaturation during apnea

In this case, we would start out by setting the relevant parameters to reflect these characteristics. In the case of the METI simulator, a scenario editor is provided so that it is not necessary to learn the precise syntax for programming scenarios. For example, instead of using a text editor to type

> events:
>> PATIENT_WEIGHT 140

we could use the scenario editor to select the "Patient Weight" parameter, then enter the amount in kilograms, and the proper syntax will be generated and saved automatically.

Following is an example scenario written for the METI simulator. It does not represent optimal coding, but rather is intended to illustrate a variety of means of achieving desired simulator responses.

```
obese_individual
baseline
{
        events:
                PATIENT_WEIGHT 140
                CHESTWALL_COM_FACTOR 0.60
                CONSO2 400.00
                PPCO2VP 60.00
                PA_CATHETER_DEPTH 0.00
                PVR_FACTOR 1.50
                RADIAL 1.00
                SF 0.10
        transitions:
}
post-induction
{
        events:
                SF 0.20
                LARYNGOSPASM 1.00
        transitions:
}
post-succinylcholine
{
        events:
                LARYNGOSPASM 0.00
                OCC_PHAR 1.00
        transitions:
}
reposition_neck
{
        events:
                OCC_PHAR 0.00
        transitions:
}
intubation
{
        events:
                administer Ephedrine 8.00
```

```
        transitions:
}
addl_anesthetic
{
        events:
                administer Ephedrine -8.00
                administer Volume -700.00
                administer Esmolol 20.00
        transitions:
}
start_surgery
{
        events:
                administer Epinephrine 20.00
                administer Volume 500.00
        transitions:
}
vagal_reflex
{
        events:
                BR_GAIN_FACTOR 4.00
                BR_MIN_PRESSURE 40.00
                SVR_FACTOR 4.00
        transitions:
}
end_vagal_reflex
{
        events:
                SVR_FACTOR 1.00
                BR_GAIN_FACTOR 1.00
                BR_MIN_PRESSURE 80.00
        transitions:
}
myocardial_ischemia
{
        events:
                ISCHEMIC_INDEX_SENS 2.00
                HR_FACTOR 1.40
        transitions:
}
NTG,_esmolol,_etc
{
        events:
                ISCHEMIC_INDEX_SENS 1.00
                HR_FACTOR 1.00
        transitions:
}
emergence
{
```

```
        events:
                HR_FACTOR 1.40
                ISCHEMIC_INDEX_SENS 1.20
        transitions:
}
extubation
{
        events:
                LARYNGOSPASM 1.00
        transitions:
}
treat_with_PPV_or_Succinylcholine
{
        events:
                LARYNGOSPASM 0.00
                administer Ephedrine 8.00
                BR_SOUND 21.00
        transitions:
}
```

The baseline state sets the initial conditions at the start of the scenario. In this case, the patient will be awake and breathing spontaneously prior to induction of anesthesia.

Chest wall compliance factor (CHESTWALL_COM_FACTOR) is reduced from 1.0 to 0.60, to simulate the effect of increased chest wall mass in an obese patient, which results in greater airway pressures during positive pressure ventilation.

To simulate the ventilation perfusion mismatching common in obese patients, oxygen consumption (CONSO2) is doubled from its default of 200 ml/min to 400, and the Shunt Fraction (SF) is increased from its default of 0.02 to 0.10. This combination results in more rapid desaturation with apnea as well as a lower arterial oxygen saturation at a given inspired oxygen concentration.

In this particular patient, we have also set the initial partial pressure of venous CO_2 (PPCO2VP) to 60 mmHg, to simulate transient respiratory depression following preoperative sedation. If desired, chronic CO_2 retention could be modelled by changing the CO_2 setpoint, so that the simulator's respiratory drive would attempt to maintain an arterial CO_2 of 60, for example.

Pulmonary vascular resistance (PVR_FACTOR) has been set to 1.5 times normal to simulate mild pulmonary hypertension. The PA_CATHETER_DEPTH and RADIAL parameters simply initialize the PA catheter as not initially inserted, but the radial artery catheter is in place so that an arterial pressure waveform can be displayed on the patient monitor.

With these changes, our new obese patient may behave approriately, but it is essential to actually test the simulation to ensure that the parameter settings are satisfactory. Frequently, some adjustments will be necessary, even if the numbers are set according to known physiology. The reason is that simulations are not perfect, and interactions may occur that result in effects that differ from expected once the hardware interfaces and respiratory gas flows come into play.

Once the parameters are set, we need to ensure that apneic desaturation occurs at rate matching clinical experience, and that inspiratory pressures are elevated to the extent expected.

With baseline parameters set, we could also save the scenario as a patient profile, so that a variety of other scenarios can be used with our morbidly obese patient.

With only these parameters set, we have a patient who should respond to anesthetic induction as a morbidly obese patient should. But because these patients are at risk for a variety of associated problems, we can create a series of problems to be managed. It is not necessary to use all the states included. Rather, we select only those which we want the trainee to manage.

A post-induction state therefore activates laryngospasm (the parameter value 1.00 turns it on), as might occur with inadequate depth and oral secretions, preventing adequate ventilation and causing rapid arterial desaturation, which is further enhanced by increasing the shunt fraction to 0.20.

When succinylcholine is given, the operator manually advances to the post-succinyl-choline state. This could also be handled automatically by including a transition test which advances to the next state if succinylcholine dose given is greater than a particular minimum dose such as 40 mg (this is actually translated internally to a blood level). Laryngospasm is turned off (parameter value 0.00), but to add a further challenger, a pharyngeal occluder has been turned on to create a difficult airway "Can't intubate" scenario. When the trainee has repositioned the head and neck appropriately or chooses an alternative intubation technique, the occluder is deflated (0.00).

With extra time elapsing for airway management, the operator makes a judgement of whether the trainee has maintained an adequate level of anesthesia for laryngoscopy and intubation. With the updated software that became available since this conference, a dose of epinephrine (10–25 mcg) would achieve the desired tachycardia and hypertension resulting from inadequate anesthesia. Likewise, subsequent administration of thiopental or another anesthetic would decrease the blood pressure and decrease sympathetic output, so that hemodynamic responses would be automatic.

At the time this scenario was written, however, the epinephrine drug model did not work appropriately. Often, we find that commercial simulators may not duplicate expected clinical responses exactly. This state therefore provides an interesting example of how we can compensate for such shortcomings. In this case, ephedrine 8 mg is administered in order to elevate the pulse rate and blood pressure appropriately. The prolonged response despite an additional dose of thiopental required further adjustments to the model, so the next state administers a *negative* dose of ephedrine to cancel the first, and also removes 700 ml of blood volume to decrease blood pressure. Esmolol is given to counteract the baroreceptor response which would otherwise increase heart rate.

At the start of surgery, epinephrine and blood volume are administered as another way to emulate endogenous catecholamine release, increasing blood pressure and heart rate.

The vagal_reflex state mimics the response to peritoneal traction. Baroreceptor gain (BR_GAIN_FACTOR) is increased from 1.0 to 4.0, resulting in a greatly enhanced fall in heart rate with an increase in mean blood pressure. The baroreceptor minimum pressure (BR_MIN_PRESSURE) in extended from the default of 80 down to 40, which expands the range of pressure over which the baroreceptor response is active. Finally, SVR_FACTOR is set to 4.0, which increases the mean blood pressure and initiates the baroreceptor-mediated fall in heart rate. The following state merely resets these values to normal to terminate the vagal reflex following cessation of surgical traction or administration of atropine.

Myocardial ischemia is created by setting the ischemic index sensitivity to its maximum and increasing heart rate by a factor of 1.4 to increase oxygen demand while decreasing diastolic time for oxygen delivery.

The ischemic episode is terminated by resetting the above parameters to their defaults when the operator manually judges that appropriate treatment has been given. Alternatively, we could have included a transition that tested for minimum doses of nitroglycerin, esmolol, etc and advanced to the resolution state automatically. While automatic transitions are easy to write when a limited number of individual drugs are each adequate when given alone, the transition becomes extremely complex when combinations of drugs act additively. In that case, you must test for different doses depending on the combinations given.

The emergence state again creates myocardial ischemia, and laryngospasm can be added upon extubation. A transition could again be used to test for a minimum dose of succinylcholine, but it would not detect continuous positive airway pressure that is often by itself adequate to break larynogospasm.

Following is another example, a short scenario that creates hypercarbia.

```
Hypercarbia
baseline
{
      events:
      transitions:
}
hypercarbia
{
      events:
            PPCO2VP 80.00 mmHg
      transitions:
}
hypercarbia_2
{
      events:
            PPCO2VP 80.00 mmHg
      transitions:
            PPCO2VP < 80.00 mmHg hypercarbia_2
}
normal_CO2
{
      events:
      transitions:
}
```

We use this scenario to simulate hypercarbia that results from an anesthesia machine fault, such as incompetent inspiratory and/or expiratory valves or depleted CO_2 absorbent. While we could anesthestize and paralyze the patient to prevent compensatory tachypnea, and then allow the simulator to be ventilated with CO_2-laden gas for a long period until arterial CO_2 concentration builds sufficiently high, the time required is impractical. Instead, we can immediately force the venous carbon dioxide partial pressure to 80 so that this scenario can follow immediately another.

However, the respiratory model will quickly drive this minor perturbation in CO_2 back down toward normal. We can overcome this by adding a recursive transition that tests for CO_2 less than 80 and keeps resetting it back up to 80.

Once the machine problem is corrected, we advance manually to the normal_CO2 scenario to allow the simulator to response normally to ventilation. The CO_2 will then return to normal gradually, dependent on alveolar ventilation.

In summary, all programmable parameters can be controlled manually during a simulation, and any scenario script can be duplicated "on-the-fly" by the operator. The real benefit of the pre-programmed scenario is the reduced time demands upon the instuctor/operator, who is then free to interact with the trainee rather than being tied to the control console. With faculty time at a premium, this can dramatically increase the amount of simulator time available to trainees.

11

ISSUES IN STARTING A SIMULATOR PROGRAM

Barry L. Zimmerman

Department of Anesthesiology
University of Rochester Medical Center
Rochester, New York 14642

1. INTRODUCTION

Acquiring a full-scale commercial anesthesia simulator will be a major investment for any program. Startup costs may well exceed the annual salary for a senior staff member, and annual maintenance costs may equal the salary of a nurse or technician. Before such an investment is undertaken, the program staff should have considered alternatives such as available personal-computer based physiologic simulations or a less capital-intensive "home-grown" system. If the decision is made to obtain a commercial system, the program should define clear objectives for the project and consider issues of space and equipment, staffing, and funding. I have prepared this brief discussion to help programs address these issues. This presentation is based primarily on our experience at the University of Rochester, and includes information about the actual costs we incurred while establishing our simulator program. Other academic institutions with similar resources have had similar experiences. The amount and type of resources that a program needs to commit to a simulator project may depend largely on local expertise; my discussion is aimed at programs which do not have staff who are already expert in computer simulations, and which will be therefore largely dependent on commercial vendors and institutional resources.

2. PROGRAM OBJECTIVES

The program should carefully define the objectives and purposes for a simulator installation. This must be done first, because the proposed uses to which the simulator will be put have a major impact on the decisions to be made about other issues such as space, personnel, and financial support. General answers such as "to enhance the educational program" are not sufficient; explicit objectives with a specific plan for accomplishing these objectives should be stated before the investment is made.

Simulators in Anesthesiology Education, edited by Henson and Lee.
Plenum Press, New York, 1998.

2.1. Teaching

The most common reason for obtaining an anesthesia simulator today is to use it as a teaching tool within a postgraduate training program in anesthesiology. This was among the earliest applications of computer simulations in anesthesiology,[1,2] and parallels work in other fields in medicine.[3,4] Computerized simulations in postgraduate training programs have produced considerable interest but have also raised questions about their ultimate utility.[5,6] Whether a computerized realistic simulation is a cost-effective means of teaching either basic or complex anesthesia skills is an issue that has not yet been resolved.

2.1.1. The program must decide if the simulator will augment teaching in the Operating Rooms (OR) (i.e., the trainee will spend the same amount of time in the OR as before) or will replace some OR experience. If the simulator will be used in "spare" time in addition to a normal day in the OR, site selection becomes very important. The facility must be located close to the OR so that both trainees and faculty have easy access. This will be discussed further in the section on selection of the facility site. If the resident (and/or teaching staff) will be removed from the OR for simulator sessions, who will cover their clinical obligations? Which will have priority, simulator training or an unanticipated (non-emergency) clinical need? If the resident (or teaching staff) will be treated like a "spare body" to be used when needed, the quality of the simulator training will probably suffer. Providing clinical coverage may involve questions of compensation and fairness that will need to be addressed before any plan is implemented.

2.1.2. If the trainee will be removed from the OR for simulator training, the facility can be distant from the OR or even off-site. If the teaching sessions will be scheduled in "non-clinical time," however, will they substitute for other didactic activities (lectures, etc.) or will they be in addition to the existing didactic program? If they are added to an existing program, will the resident (and staff) be expected to give up personal time (evenings, weekends, etc.)? If the simulator will substitute for some part of the didactic program, which parts will be eliminated?

2.2. Evaluation

Evaluation of professional skills is one of the more problematic areas in simulator use. Before it can be used as an effective tool for performance evaluation, it must be *validated* against other commonly accepted tools for summative evaluation. This validation has not yet been done for evaluation of clinical anesthesia skills. Dr. Robert Helmreich[7] pointed out at this meeting that it was several decades after flight simulation was used as an educational tool that it became accepted as a tool for performance evaluation. While the process may take somewhat less time now, it is still reasonable to assume that a period of years will pass before the profession accepts electronic simulators as equal to, or even complementary to, traditional written and oral examinations and observation of performance by a skilled practitioner. The American Board of Anesthesiology has considered the use of simulators in its certification process, but as of the spring of 1997 has concluded that the technology has not yet been sufficiently developed or validated to serve as a tool for the Board's use.[8] The program director must consider the possibility that a resident who has been given an unsatisfactory report on the basis of simulator-based evaluation might make a claim against the program for "arbitrary" action, based on the lack of data suggesting that the simulator is a valid evaluation tool. For the present time, the use of a simulator for performance evaluation within an anesthesiology program should be approached with caution. However, research in this area should be encouraged.

2.3. Staff Continuing Medical Education (CME)

One of the more important applications of simulator technology might be for anesthesia staff CME. Again, the situation is analogous to the airline industry, where pilots are required to "re-qualify" in simulators periodically. Simulators are most useful for practicing skills used only rarely, or for the initial experience in new situations or with new techniques. It has already been suggested that practicing anesthesiologists should go through "refresher courses" in the management of simulated anesthetic crises on a regular basis.[9] Also, the staff's initial experience with a new drug or monitor might be with a simulated patient.

2.4. Research

Simulator technology and application would appear to be a very fruitful area for research projects in many disciplines. The most promising areas would include both research into the simulator technology itself, and research in other areas that might use a simulator as a tool.

2.4.1. Despite considerable work in this field, much research remains to be done before the simulator's role is defined as a tool for teaching or evaluation. As mentioned previously, studies that compare the results of simulator-based performance evaluation to other standard measures of competence will be needed before the simulator can be used to replace or even complement existing methodology. Since these studies will of necessity be longitudinal, several years will be needed to obtain even limited data.

2.4.2. The simulator can also be used as a tool for investigating other subjects. When clear performance criteria can be defined, the simulator could be used as an environment for studying the effect of various factors on task performance. For instance, Denisco *et al* have used "simulations" (but not simulators) to investigate the effect of sleep deprivation on performance of anesthetic tasks.[10] The simulator would appear to be an ideal tool for such studies. Simulations have also been used to evaluate the impact of new technologies like "smart alarms" on the anesthesiologist's ability to respond to critical situations.[11]

2.4.3. Resident Recruiting. The value of having a simulator for attracting residents into a program must be considered highly speculative. At the present time there is no evidence that applicants take the presence of a simulator into account when choosing a program. Based on our own experience at the University of Rochester, many other factors appear to be more important in the decision process. If a program wishes to allocate resources to improving resident recruiting, it may want to consider spending the money on program improvement or faculty development.

2.5. Entrepreneurial Activities

Anesthesia simulators have some potential as sources for additional income for an institution or program, but the approach to all of the issues regarding starting a simulator program may be very different if commercial profit is one of the goals. The impact of using a simulator facility for income generation will be discussed further in the sections regarding each of the issues.

3. FACILITIES AND EQUIPMENT

3.1. Simulator Site

The choice of location for the simulator will be determined by multiple factors. Probably the most relevant factor in most programs will be the availability of suitable space. To make the simulator program practical, however, several factors should be considered. If the main purpose of the facility is to train clinical residents with clinical faculty, the simulator should be near the OR suite. This will allow both staff and the trainees to have access to the simulator at whatever times during the day that they are free. This may for brief periods at odd times in the day. If the simulator is located off-site or at a distance from the OR, there may not be enough time to prepare the simulator, teach a scenario, debrief, and shut down in the time available. Also, technical support, supplies, equipment, and items such as piped gases may be more readily available near the OR.

If a simulator program is to be used primarily for training non-OR staff or outside visitors, or for research, and especially if there will be dedicated non-clinical teaching staff, an off-site location is more reasonable. In these cases the installation could be located in an area distant from the OR suite, so that simulator activities would not interfere with clinical operations.

When considering available sites for a simulator installation, the program should consider the subject of "ownership." If the program "owns" (in the sense of controls) the site, it has more flexibility to remodel and install additional items such as video equipment. Also, the program will be able to dispose of the facility if other needs require it. If the facility is set up in "borrowed" space, the owner may restrict the programs ability to "customize" the space, and may evict the program for any reason. If the program cannot obtain actual ownership of the site, a firm commitment amounting to a lease should be sought, including the requirement for suitable advance notification of eviction, and clearly defining what modifications the program may make in the facility.

3.2. Support Space

A single room containing the simulator is not an optimal setting for the project, unless the objectives are very limited. Additional space for storage, debriefing, control, observation, and related activities should be available. If the simulator sessions are to be observed by others as part of routine operations, suitable provisions must be made to ensure that observers do not disrupt or influence the scenario. Observation through a window (one-way glass is optimal) or by video monitors will allow discussion as the scenario progresses. If the observers are in the simulator room, they should maintain silence until the scenario ends. An additional "teaching" room with chairs, a table, whiteboard, projection screen, etc., would provide an area to permit relaxed discussion either before or after a session, or for related teaching activities. If the simulator room is not in the OR suite, there must be storage space available for supplies, spare parts, and other items that may be used in special scenarios. The operator controlling the simulation, if different from the teaching staff, must be located in such a way that the control functions will not interfere with the scenario. A separate control room is probably a luxury in most cases, but increases the flexibility and ease of use for the operators.

4. PERSONNEL

4.1. Project Director/Team Leader

There should be one person given overall leadership of the project. The selection of this person will depend in large part on the planned uses of the simulator. Computer skills are not absolutely essential, but the team leader should have skills appropriate to the planned utilization. If the simulator is to be used primarily for teaching, the leader should be a teacher, and so forth. It is not necessary that this person should be an anesthesiologist, or even a physician. It could be a nurse, a non-physician scientist, or even a technician. If the program were not going to recruit a dedicated director for the simulator project, it would be reasonable to compensate the leader in some way, usually by providing time at program expense (e.g., by providing coverage for his/her other duties). The program should consider if it is cost-effective to allow a clinical anesthesiologist to do this, or if it might actually be more efficient to hire someone else. In any event, the leader should be interested in the project and be willing to put in the time required.

4.2. Teaching Faculty

A small "core" group of teaching faculty should be selected from an identified pool of volunteers. The teaching staff should be chosen in consultation with the project director. Teaching staff could be physicians or other interested and capable staff. If they are clinical faculty, they will need to be given time to participate. Other compensation would be at the discretion of the program director, and might depend on the sources of funding for the project (see below).

4.3. Technical Staff

A simulator program requires considerable technical support. If the simulator is going to be used for significant periods of time on a daily basis, a dedicated technician is appropriate. Otherwise, a small number of technicians (two or three) should be designated to form the support team for the simulator. This allows sharing of responsibilities and prevents interruption in services when one person is unavailable, but keeps the training needs limited to a small group. Background experience could be in any technical field, but computer experience is useful because of the need to do software installation and maintenance. Factory training is available from the major vendors, and is mandatory for anyone who will be working inside the hardware.

4.4. Support Staff (Office)

Even a small program will require some office support. A secretary would be needed to send out notification of teaching sessions, generate personnel and facilities schedules, and maintain correspondence with the simulator vendor. If the simulator program is to be considered a "cost center" or used for revenue generation, bookkeeping or accounting support may be needed. If the simulator is to be used in a program for performance evaluation, secure and confidential records must be maintained. Again, the size of the program and available funds will determine if office staff will be dedicated to the simulator program or existing office personnel will be used.

5. SOURCES OF FUNDING

5.1. Private Practice Income

If a simulator is to be used in the context of a clinical training program, much of the initial support for a simulator program may well come from funds obtained from practice revenue. Much of this support will be in the form of "volunteer" time put in by the teaching faculty, even if the simulator itself is purchased by the institution. If the program assigns staff from other activities to allow the teaching staff to have time out of the OR, this amounts to a direct subsidy of the simulator program from practice funds.

5.2. Institutional Funds

The university or hospital may wish to contribute to the purchase or operation of a simulator facility. This probably would require making the simulator available to other programs within the institution, rather than a single department. For instance, a Department of Anesthesiology might offer to train the staff in other departments in airway management, conscious sedation, or hemodynamic monitoring. If the institution itself does not wish to participate, the sponsoring department might want to contact other programs to see if there is interest in collaboration. Programs that have expressed interest in simulator training in Rochester have included Emergency Medicine, Critical Care and Surgery. Entering into a collaborative agreement with the institution or other departments will place demands on the facility that may conflict with those of the primary department. It is essential to have centralized accounting and scheduling for a joint simulator program, and the role of the project director becomes even more important.

5.3. Research Grants

Projects involving investigators with the skills and interests needed to generate formal research protocols and grant applications should seek external funding. In addition to major funding sources, anesthesiologists should consider sources such as the Foundation for Anesthesia Education and Research (FAER) and the Anesthesia Patient Safety Foundation (APSF). Local funds may also be available. The University of Rochester offers "Innovations in Patient Care Grants" to clinical staff who are seeking ways of improving quality or efficiency of health care in the hospital.

5.4. Corporate Grants

One of the most important uses for simulators in the near future may well be as a means of introducing clinical staff to new drugs, equipment, or procedures. In these cases, funds would probably be available from the companies who have an interest in putting their product before the professional staff in a safe, controlled, and efficient manner. At the University of Rochester, we have used our simulator to train anesthesia providers in the use of new narcotic analgesics, supported in part by funds from the pharmaceutical company. If such an arrangement is sought, however, the program should keep in mind that such support usually includes a need for contractual agreements that might be very restrictive. Any restrictions or obligations placed on the program need to be explicitly stated and carefully reviewed, probably by legal counsel.

Table 1. Real and potential program startup costs at the University of Rochester (1994 U.S. dollars)

	Actual cost	Potential cost
Purchase	150,000	
Installation	38,500	
Construction		
Nitrogen	1,000	
Regulators	800	
Machine		35,000
Monitor		35,000

6. VENTURE CAPITAL

If the simulator program is intended to generate revenue, investment income from private sources can provide some funding. However, this puts an even higher burden of responsibility on the program providers than does an institutional collaboration or corporate grants. Strict accounting practices will be necessary, and both legal and financial advisers should carefully review any contractual agreements.

7. STARTUP COSTS

The actual and potential costs for starting the anesthesia simulator program at the University of Rochester in 1994 are shown in Table 1. Actual costs are the real amounts paid for the items; potential costs were avoided by making use of equipment loaned by the respective manufacturers. The purchase price included all equipment, computer hardware, and software, but no maintenance beyond the initial warranty. The simulator vendor did all hardware installation. Site construction costs were limited to installing nitrogen gas lines into the simulator room, and the purchase and installation of pressure regulators for the various gas supply tanks and lines. The anesthesia machine and physiologic monitors were obtained on loan as "demo" units from their respective manufacturers. Estimated costs for purchase of these units are presented in the "potential" column.

8. OPERATING COSTS

Table 2 shows the actual costs for operating and maintaining the simulator at the University of Rochester in 1995. The manufacturer's service contract was for one year of on-site service and software and hardware upgrades. Routine preventive maintenance was not included. We do not have a full-time technician assigned to the simulator project; the

Table 2. First-year operating costs at the University of Rochester (1995 U.S. dollars)

	Real costs	Potential cost
Contract	11,688	
Tech staff	14,000	
Supplies	1,000	
Faculty	?	50,000
Other (VCR, etc.)		?

expense for technical support represents an estimate of the amount of work done by an anesthesia technician for maintenance, setup, routine service, installing updated hardware and software, and assisting the teaching faculty during sessions. Using outdated or used supplies and drugs minimized expenses for disposable and expendable supplies.

Faculty support was provided voluntarily. The teaching faculty were not compensated or reimbursed for the time spent working with the simulator. The estimate for faculty time was based on our need for about one-third of a faculty FTE to support the simulator.

REFERENCES

1. Schwid HA: A flight simulator for general anesthesia training. Computers and Biomedical Research 20:64–75, 1987.
2. Gaba DM, DeAnda A: A comprehensive anesthesia simulation environment: re-creating the operating room for research and training. Anesthesiology 69:387–394, 1988.Byrne AJ, Hilton PJ, Lunn JN: Basic simulations for anaesthetists. A pilot study of the ACCESS system. Anaesthesia 49:376–381, 1994.
3. Miller MD: Simulations in medical education: a review. Medical Teacher 9:35–41, 1987.
4. Stillman PL, Swanson DB, Smee S: Assessing the clinical skills of residents with standardized patients. Ann Intern Med 105:762–771, 1986.
5. Gravenstein JS: Training devices and simulators [ed]. Anesthesiology 69:295–297, 1988.
6. Asbury AJ: Simulators for general anaesthesia. Br J Anaesth 73:285–286, 1994.
7. Helmreich R: Personal communication.
8. Rosenthal M: Personal communication.
9. Schwid HA, O'Donnell D: Anesthesiologists' management of simulated critical incidents. Anesthesiology 76:495–501, 1992.
10. Denisco RA, Drummond JN, Gravenstein JS: The effect of fatigue on the performance of a simulated anesthetic monitoring task. J Clin Monit 3:22–24, 1987.
11. Westenskow DR, Orr JA, Simon FH, Ing D, Bender H-J, Frankenberger H: Intelligent alarms reduce anesthesiologist's response time to critical faults. Anesthesiology 77:1074–1079, 1992.

RESEARCH TECHNIQUES IN HUMAN PERFORMANCE USING REALISTIC SIMULATION

David M. Gaba[1,2]

[1]VA Palo Alto HCS
[2]Department of Anesthesiology
Stanford University

1. REALISTIC SIMULATION AS A RESEARCH TOOL

This chapter concerns the research uses of realistic patient simulators in the evaluation of different aspects of human performance of clinical personnel. The issues of human performance in health care and patient safety may be viewed as a jigsaw puzzle for which at least three different experimental approaches can provide interlocking, and complementary pieces. No single approach can give the entire picture of human error and safety. Realistic simulation has many advantages and some disadvantages for research. I believe that high-fidelity realistic simulations of patient care situations are an important tool in studying error modalities in high criticality health care environments. These environments include anesthesia, intensive care, emergency and trauma care, labor and delivery, cardiac catheterization laboratories, and cardiac arrest teams. I first discuss how simulation fits in the jigsaw puzzle with other research techniques for investigating human performance.

1.1. Retrospective Reports as an Information Source

The first technique is assembling *retrospective reports* describing either minor or serious events. This has the advantage of dealing with *real events* in their actual organizational context and, if desired, *serious events*. However, retrospective reporting has many limitations, whether it is done for a special study or as part of routine quality management. Reluctance to "self-report" means that many cases go unreported in which errors did occur. This creates a major selection bias concerning the cases that are reported. The data available from retrospective reports are often scant or flawed. Reliable information about what actually occurred is limited, since even the immediate recollection of case events by participants is full of gaps, inconsistencies and biases. Although automated electronic data management systems may add additional reliable retrospective information they cannot

Simulators in Anesthesiology Education, edited by Henson and Lee.
Plenum Press, New York, 1998.

provide information about the activities of the clinicians and their interaction with each other. It is for this reason, for example, that commercial aviation uses both a flight *data* recorder and a cockpit *voice* recorder to reconstruct aviation accidents.

1.2. Observation of Actual Patient Care as an Information Source

The observation of actual *patient care in progress* (by an observer or a camera) also deals with *real cases*, and permits collecting as much *prospective data* as possible. Especially if audio and video recordings are made, the data can be unbiased and archival. The main disadvantage of this technique is that serious patient care problems requiring significant intervention by clinicians will arise unpredictably and infrequently (compared to total patient care time), so that most of what is observed will be relatively mundane. There are limits to how much data can actually be acquired without intruding excessively on patient care or the privacy of patients and staff. Finally, when analyzing real cases either retrospectively or prospectively, the exact *cause* of the events observed may never be known, so that each case contains a unique set of circumstances which may never be repeated. The inter-individual variability of error occurrence and error mechanisms cannot be investigated.

1.3. Advantages of Realistic Simulation as an Information Source

Simulation, by contrast, offers the advantages of *prospective* and *repeated* observation of the response to *serious events* whose *etiology and timing are known with certainty*. This is done with absolute safety to patients (since none are involved) and dispenses with the need to recruit patient subjects. The hallmarks of simulation studies are their *controllability* and *reproducibility* (at least in comparison to studies of real cases). If desired, scenarios can be designed to modulate important underlying variables such as complexity, time pressure, and stress. Entire teams can undergo testing or else various team members can be played by knowledgeable actors so as to probe the abilities of a sub-component of the overall team. The environment allows collection of relatively intrusive archival data (computer files, multiple video views, and high quality audio recording) without intruding on actual patient care. Similarly, other intrusive techniques are possible including alterations in availability of clinical data or data formats on monitors.

In general, experiments on current patient simulators can be highly reproducible. To the extent that all "events" are pre-defined and instantiated by the simulator, each subject will see the same underlying phenomena. Of course, once a subject begins to treat the patient, the further evolution of the clinical situation will change relative to other subjects whose treatment is different. One can present essentially the same scenario to different individuals at different times.

A further advantage of simulation is that the investigator can allow errors to occur which, if observed during a real case, would require immediate intervention to protect the patient. Thus, one can observe the complete spectrum of human performance of different clinicians without providing a patient safety net. If performance is sub-optimal the cascading results of the errors will be observed to their ultimate conclusion.

1.4. Disadvantages of Simulation as an Information Source

The chief disadvantage of simulation is that *it is not, and never can be, entirely real.* Existing patient simulators are imperfect (although still relatively high fidelity). Current medical knowledge is vastly inferior to that present in aerodynamics and aviation. Simulators involve many compromises and approximations. The most fundamental is the patient mannequin which can never re-create the subtleties of the human body. Mathematical models of physiology and pharmacology are incomplete and approximate. Nonetheless, imperfect simulator fidelity is probably not the greatest disadvantage to simulation as a research tool The greatest disadvantage is that subjects know they are working under scrutiny in a simulator environment. This tends to make them hypervigilant, but they may also sometimes act with a "cavalier" attitude knowing that no real patient is at risk. Thus, although the physical clinical environment can be re-created with some accuracy (although the clinical equipment in use may not match that most familiar to a particular research subject), one cannot fully re-create the organizational structure of the clinical setting or the subject's real "motivational" setting. Such factors probably play a large role in the performance of clinicians and the artificial simulation environment cannot fully capture these factors adequately.

From a practical standpoint there are some countermeasures to the hypervigilance that can occur during simulations. One is to inform the subject of the possibility of some "null scenarios" in which nothing very exciting happens. By so warning subjects, and by using some null scenarios, they become aware of the real dangers of overreacting as well as underreacting to problems. A similar countermeasure is to use long scenarios in which there are no significant events for substantial portions of the case. We also believe that to some degree the complacency induced by the obvious fact that a real patient's life is *not* at stake will counteract some of the hypervigilance. As a general rule, we have argued that while the exact events of each subject's performance might or might not happen the same way for that subject if the situation occurred in a real case, the performance is representative of events that will certainly occur to some practitioners faced with the same situation.

1.5. Experience with Realistic Simulation as a Research Tool

My own laboratory has studied anesthesiologists managing simulated patients in a realistic hands-on simulator with and without critical perioperative events.[1-5] More recently we have begun studying intensive care unit clinicians (nurses and physicians) during simulations of ICU situations. We have previously reported on the kinds of errors made by anesthesiologists during simulations, both in response to the scenarios presented and the unplanned errors they created on their own. Outright vigilance failures were rare - some manifestation of a problem was usually detected fairly quickly. Vigilant detection did not however guarantee the rapid implementation of appropriate therapies. Regardless of the level of experience (including faculty and private practitioners) there was at least one "catastrophic" failure in each experience group. Fixation errors were common[6]. This is the *persistent* failure to revise a diagnosis or plan in the face of readily available evidence that suggests a revision is necessary. Unplanned errors were also common[3]. These were errors triggered *de novo* by clinicians while managing a critical situation presented by the experimenter. These data, as well as data from real clinical situations have been extremely useful for defining models of clinician cognition[7-9] and of accident evolution[10-12]. Similar results have come from studying anesthesiologists managing simulated situations on a computer-screen simulator[13].

Therefore, simulations clearly give an unique view on error modes and the inter-individual differences between clinicians managing nearly identical situations. Such views cannot be obtained in any other way. Thus, I believe that simulation studies should be an integral part of the study of clinician performance in a variety clinical environments, but these data *must* be combined with data from similar techniques applied to real patient care in which the disadvantages of simulation do not apply[14,15]. By combining data from settings the unique advantages of each can be utilized while minimizing the disadvantages.

2. MEASUREMENT TECHNIQUES FOR HUMAN PERFORMANCE RESEARCH

Most of the techniques that can be used in simulation studies are similar to or identical to those that can be used to investigate performance in real work situations. The literature on these techniques is massive; this chapter can only provide a very brief introduction to a few of them. The reader should consult standard references[16,17] and the research literature on human factors for additional information. I have also indicated where well-known investigators in anesthesiology have been applying these techniques. Interested new investigators may wish to contact the experienced investigators for advice.

2.1. Measurements of "Mental Workload," "Vigilance," and "Attention"

Many studies focus on the measurement of performance issues related to "mental workload", "vigilance", "attention", and perhaps the lack thereof (as in fatigue studies). These concepts are readily understood, but not so readily defined in an operational sense for experiment. The types of measures of workload and attention are shown in Table 1 and described below.

Table 1. Measures of workload

Physiologic measures
  Heart rate and heart rate variability
  Eye tracking (measure of visual attentiveness)
  EEG/Evoked potentials (difficult in anesthesia because subjects are moving)

Primary task measures
  Increase workload of main (clinical) task until a performance failure is detected (this can only be performed during simulations)

Secondary task measures (most commonly utilized)
  Loading paradigm: Increase workload of a mandatory second task until performance failure occurs on the main task. This indicates how much workload the main task demands. This can only be performed during simulations.
  Probing paradigm: Add a relatively non-intrusive second task. Instruct that the primary task always takes precedence and measure the performance on the secondary task. This performance is an inverse measure of "workload" or "spare capacity" since the subject can only attend to the secondary task when not fully loaded by the first. When the secondary task occurs infrequently and/or involves subtle cues this becomes more like a traditional test of "vigilance"

Subjective workload measures (how much workload the subject or observer perceives)
  Retrospective questionnaire (after completion of work)
  Concurrent assessment (during work)
    By anesthetist
    By observer
  Note: Multiple sub-scales of subjective workload can be assessed, but existing data have shown a high concordance between them during anesthesia care. Also, the observer and anesthetist scores also correlate highly.

2.1.1. Physiologic Measures. Some measures rely on the human body itself to give evidence of the mental workload encountered. Heart rate is related to workload, and more specifically certain frequency components of heart rate variability have been linked to mental workload[18]. Thus, with the correct analysis, Holter-type monitoring of personnel can allow measurements of mental workload. Matt Weinger (UCSD), among others has been attempting these types of measurements in anesthesiology.

Eye gaze is a fairly direct measure of visual attention (although it is possible to be looking at something while not seeing it). Thus, eye tracking systems which can continuously identify where the gaze is directed can provide good data on visual attention. Per Foege Jensen in Denmark (Herlev Hospital) has had some experience with attempting to apply eye tracking systems in anesthesia. These systems are expensive and cumbersome, and it is not clear whether they can be applied successfully to anesthesiology. It is important to note however that techniques that might be too intrusive to be practical in the real OR might be usable in the simulator environment.

Considerable research has been done on EEG measures, especially evoked potentials, as signs of mental workload[18]. However, essentially all of these studies have taken place with subjects seated at a workstation or cockpit-like setting. Such systems are even more expensive and cumbersome than are eye-tracking systems. However, they might be applicable in the simulation environment for certain types of studies. The EEG and EOG (electrooculogram) can be useful for assessing sleepiness and whether a subject has actually fallen asleep, and might be applicable to simulation studies of fatigued vs. rested subjects. Steve Howard at VA Palo Alto/Stanford University has experience with this application of EEG/EOG measurements.

2.1.2. Primary Task Measures. In this technique to assess workload the performance of the subject is measured on a typical set of work tasks (the primary task). The primary task is made more complex (increased load) until the performance of the subject starts to decrease. This level of load is assumed to be the maximum workload the subject is capable of handling at that time. One problem with such an approach in anesthesiology is that the primary task of patient care is extremely complex and thus it is difficult to measure performance quantitatively. For patient care, one might find sub-tasks for which performance can be quantitated. If so, the primary task loading paradigm to measure workload capacity might be feasible. Again, the simulator environment would allow one to increase the clinical complexity ad infinitum even to the level of serious degradation of care.

2.1.3. Secondary Task Measures. A secondary task is a task additional to the primary work task. The secondary task may be totally separate from the work (e.g. answering addition problems while conducting an anesthetic). Alternatively (and with greater difficulty) secondary tasks can be grafted onto components of the primary task. When this is done the secondary tasks is called an *embedded task*. For example, if a subject is asked to identify when specific numeric values of vital signs occur, this would be a secondary task embedded in the primary task which already includes watching the vital signs. There are two different ways in which secondary tasks can be used to assess workload. One is called secondary task "loading", in which the complexity of the primary work task is kept constant, but the load of the secondary task is increased until the performance on the primary task fails. As for primary task measures this requires that performance on the primary task be quantifiable.

The more common technique for using secondary tasks is in the "probing" methodology. In this method the secondary task is usually a very simple one. In anesthesia secondary tasks have included performing simple arithmetic problems[19], identifying when a red light illuminates near the patient monitor display[20], or identifying special alphanumeric sequences on a patient monitor display[21]. Subjects are instructed that the primary task takes precedence over the secondary task. Then, the performance on the secondary task becomes a measure of the "spare capacity" to deal with it while simultaneously maintaining performance on the primary task. Such measures of "spare capacity" can be seen as measures of "vigilance". This is especially true when the incidence rate of the secondary task probes is relatively low (i.e. infrequent) and relatively random.

Secondary task measures of spare capacity and vigilance have been used by Gaba and Lee at VA Palo Alto / Stanford[19], Weinger et al (UCSD in collaboration with Gaba)[20], and Loeb, et al (Dr. Loeb was at UC Davis but is now at U Arizona Tucson)[21–23] for studying anesthesiologists.

2.1.4. Subjective Workload Measures. Perhaps the simplest means of assessing workload is to ask the subjects how loaded they feel. Subjective assessment of workload is an important adjunct to objective measures. Even if one can manage the workload, if it is subjectively difficult it will lead to fatigue and anxiety over the long run. Conversely, it may be important to demonstrate when workload is too high to be managed even when the subject feels "OK", for this may suggest complacency. Traditionally, subjects filled out a questionnaire about the workload of a "session" after it was completed. However, such retrospective assessment cannot track the ebb and flow of workload during complex and time-varying situations. Other investigators have used concurrent rating of workload, both by the subject and by the investigator[20]. There are dozens of workload assessment scales. Some use multiple separate axes of workload components, but for anesthesiologists it has been shown that the concordance between the axes is very high, so that a single question about overall workload is probably as useful as asking about multiple axes[19,20].

2.2. Performance Measures

It would be highly desirable to measure the *performance* of anesthesiologists, and to compare performance under different conditions. Unfortunately, as suggested above, patient care is a very complex task for which performance cannot be easily quantitated. There have been several approaches to attempting to measure performance

2.2.1. Task Analysis. The approach in task analysis is to break up the complex task of patient care into the minute sub-tasks that are actually performed. This is a standard technique of human factors engineering. By looking at what sub-tasks are performed, in what order, and how long is spent on each, one can distinguish, to some degree between experienced and novice anesthetists. Task analysis data provide a foundation of objective information about the work that can underlay more complex performance assessments. Considerable work on task analysis has been done by Weinger, et al.[20] To date, nearly all task analysis work in anesthesiology has looked at the tasks of a single anesthetist (e.g. resident or CRNA) but has largely ignored the distribution of tasks between that individual and others (attending, assisting anesthetist, etc.). Gaba and Weinger are in the process of analyzing task distribution and coordination between multiple anesthetists.

2.2.2. Technical Performance ("Correct" Diagnosis and Therapy). Much of what we intuitively think of as "performance" of anesthetists has to do with the accomplishment of key technical actions of patient care. Intraoperatively this largely means diagnosing and treating anticipated or unanticipated clinical situations, as well as the execution of the standard actions of the chosen anesthetic plan.

One can measure this "technical performance" in a variety of ways discussed below. The simulator gives a major advantage over real cases in assessing technical performance because with the simulator one knows for sure the nature of the underlying problem. This allows one to define in advance the kinds of technical responses which are appropriate, neutral or inappropriate. In real cases one must conjecture from the clinical data what is the underlying problem, and this is often difficult. A further advantage of the simulator is that each subject will face nearly the same situation, allowing differences between subjects to become manifest in ways that would be masked by differences in the clinical situation in real cases.

Technical performance can be measured first by assessing the response time to different aspects of diagnosis and treatment[1-3,13]. In the simulator the time an event is triggered is known precisely, as is the time of appearance of various clinical manifestations. Thus, one can measure the response time to:

- Detecting the existence of the problem
- Diagnosing the nature and/or exact cause of the problem
- Beginning any of several possible treatments for the problem
- Completing therapy of the problem (to whatever threshold is desired)

One can also record the diagnostic modalities or sources of information used to diagnose and manage a specific problem[1,2].

In addition to response time and information sources– which can be measured with reasonable precision (although there can be some arguments as to what constitutes making a diagnosis or completing therapy) – one can measure the *correctness* of the diagnosis and therapy, the appropriateness of the sequence of activities, and the occurrence of any "*errors*" in diagnosis and management. But these measures are even more subjective than are the response times. It is either necessary to prepare careful operational definitions of correctness (which can always be challenged) or to use a panel of experts to rate individually or by consensus the correctness of the actions taken. While there is likely a greater degree of interrater reliability concerning technical matters than "behavioral matters", the reliability of subjective ratings of correctness of diagnosis and therapy has not yet been determined in anesthesia.

A variety of methods for assessing technical performance in simulations have been described by Gaba, Schwid, Chopra, and Jensen [1-3,13,24]

2.2.3. Behavioral Performance. Several groups involved with simulators believe strongly that technical performance is only one (essential) component of good patient care. The other is manifesting appropriate patient care "behaviors" that promote optimal technical work and team coordination. To a large degree these groups have drawn from the extensive assessment of cockpit management behaviors of airline pilots, although the principle of evaluating patient care behavior is independent of this analogy.

The particular behaviors one believes are important will depend on the underlying model of optimal individual and team cognition during complex patient care situations.

There are at least two methods for analyzing behaviors. One is to conduct formal quantitative (and qualitative) linguistic analyses of the utterances of the personnel. This technique has been used by several investigators in aviation to evaluate the behavioral performance of cockpit crews[25-27].

However, not all behaviors are manifested through utterances. A more common technique is to use "anchored" subjective ratings of behavior on several axes of interest. The ratings are anchored by giving definitions for each point on the rating scale, and by training of raters as to what constitutes each level of performance. Some examples are shown in table 2 below. For several years, the NASA/University of Texas Aerospace Crew Performance Project has been producing anchored subjective rating scales for Crew Resource Management behaviors in aviation.[28-31] These have been adapted by two groups (VA Palo Alto / Stanford and the University of Basel) in anesthesia for use in evaluating anesthesia resource management behaviors. The evaluation of interrater reliability and predictive power of these scales is still in progress and it is not yet known how well they will work.

Table 2. Example of subjective anchored ratings for one marker of crisis management behaviors

Marker 5: Leadership/Followership	Phase 1:	0	1	2	3	4	5
	Phase 2:	0	1	2	3	4	5

Note: This marker addresses the overall performance of the crew as a whole.

Leader:
- The "hot seat" anesthetist takes command or delegates command to more qualified associate.
- Help is called for as necessary; errs on side of calling for help.
- The leader acts decisively (e.g. commits to declare emergency early vs. late).
- Coordinates activities of all crew; checks with crew about task status.
- Stays free to direct except when necessary.

Followers:
- Identify the leader clearly.
- Respond promptly; report task status periodically.
- Work through leader most of time; exert leadership as necessary to backup "hot seat" anesthetist.

Comments:

Anchor points for ratings

0. Not observed

    Few if any examples of performance related to this marker were observed during the phase being rated.

1. Poor performance

    There is a *noted absence of effective behaviors* and/or a *substantial presence of detrimental behaviors* which together markedly impair satisfactory patient management. The performance is significantly below that expected for an average crew of experienced practitioners. An explanation for this rating is mandatory.

2. Sub-standard (minimally acceptable) performance:

    While there is sufficient effective behavior to carry out acceptable patient management the *behaviors are weak* or *enough detrimental behaviors occur* such that management is less effective than would be expected from an average crew of experienced practitioners.

3. Standard performance:

    The preponderance of behaviors are reasonably effective and there are *only occasional or fewer weak or detrimental behaviors*. Crisis management behavior is what would be expected from an average crew of experienced practitioners.

4. Good performance:

    There is a *preponderance of effective behaviors* with some strong or exceptional behaviors which particularly promote and maintain crew performance. *Weak or detrimental behaviors are rare*. The crisis management behavior is better than would be expected from an average crew of experienced practitioners.

5. Excellent performance:

    Nearly all behaviors are strong with frequent examples of *exceptional crisis management skill*. Weak or detrimental behaviors are rare or nonexistent. The crew's behavior serves as a model for teamwork—truly noteworthy and effective. An explanation is mandatory.

Preliminary data from my own laboratory[32] suggests that in spite of careful training of raters, there is still substantial inter-rater variance, a large portion of which seems to come from the difficulty in aggregating complex behaviors *over time* into a single rating score. For example, in rating communication during management of an anesthetic crisis (e.g. MH) the team might be communicating well at one instant only to be communicating poorly the next. Aggregating these differing behaviors, even over a 5–15 minute period, will vary between raters. At present it seems reasonable to suggest that the combination of at least two raters would be necessary to eliminate biased results.

3. SUMMARY

Investigating human performance is challenging in all settings. The simulator environment offers substantial advantages relative to real clinical cases. Many techniques of standard human factors research have been adapted by different research groups for use in analyzing human performance in anesthesiology. This overview should help new investigators get a sense of the different possibilities that might be suitable for their research.

REFERENCES

1. Gaba DM , DeAnda A: The response of anesthesia trainees to simulated critical incidents. Anesth Analg 68: 444–451, 1989.
2. DeAnda A, Gaba DM: The role of experience in the response to simulated critical incidents. Anesth Analg 72: 308–315, 1991.
3. DeAnda A, Gaba DM: Unplanned incidents during comprehensive anesthesia simulation. Anesth Analg 71: 77–82, 1990.
4. Botney R, Gaba DM, Howard SK, Jump B: The role of fixation error in preventing the detection and correction of a simulated volatile anesthetic overdose (abstract). Anesthesiology 79: A1115, 1993.
5. Botney R, Gaba DM, Howard SK: Anesthesiologist performance during a simulated loss of pipeline oxygen (abstract). Anesthesiology 79: A1118, 1993.
6. De Keyser V, Woods DD: Fixation errors: Failures to revise situation assessment in dynamic and risky systems, Systems Reliability Assessment. Edited by Colombo AG, Saiz de Bustamonte A. Boston, Kluwer Academic Publishers, 1990, pp 231–251 .
7. Gaba DM: Dynamic decision-making in anesthesiology: cognitive models and training approaches, Advanced Models of Cognition for Medical Training and Practice. Edited by Evans DA, Patel VL. Berlin, Springer-Verlag, 1992, pp 122–147 .
8. Gaba DM: Human error in dynamic medical environments, Human Error in Medicine. Edited by Bogner MS. Hillsdale, NJ, Lawrence Erlbaum Associates, 1994, pp 197–224 .
9. Gaba DM, Howard SK, Small S: Situation awareness in Anesthesiology. Hum Factors 37: 20–31, 1995.
10. Gaba DM, Maxwell M, DeAnda A: Anesthetic mishaps: breaking the chain of accident evolution. Anesthesiology 66: 670–676, 1987.
11. Gaba DM: Human error in anesthetic mishaps. Int Anesthesiol Clin 27: 137–147, 1989.
12. Gaba DM: Human Performance Issues in Anesthesia Patient Safety. Probs Anesth 5: 329–350, 1991.
13. Schwid HA, O'Donnell D: Anesthesiologists' management of simulated critical incidents. Anesthesiology 76: 495–501, 1992.
14. Mackenzie CF, Hu PF, Horst RL, Group LOTAS: An audio-video acquisition system for automated data acquisition in the clinical environment. J Clin Monit 11: 335–341, 1995.
15. Mackenzie CF, Martin P, Xiao Y: Video analysis of uncorrected esophageal intubation. Anesthesiology 84: 1494–1503, 1996.
16. Boff KR, Kaufman L, Thomas JP: Handbook of perception and human performance. New York, Wiley-Interscience, 1986.
17. Salvendy G: Handbook of human factors. New York, Wiley-Interscience, 1987.
18. O'Donnell RD, Eggemeier FT: Workload assessment methodology, Handbook of Perception and Human Performance . Edited by Boff KR, Kaufman L, Thomas JP. New York, Wiley Interscience, 1986, pp 42–49.
19. Gaba DM, Lee T: Measuring the workload of the anesthesiologist. Anesth Analg 71: 354–361, 1990.

20. Weinger MB, Herndon OW, Zornow MH, Paulus MP, Gaba DM, Dallen LT: An objective methodology for task analysis and workload assessment in anesthesia providers. Anesthesiology 77–92, 1994.
21. Loeb RG: A measure of intraoperative attention to monitor displays. Anesth Analg 76: 337–341, 1993.
22. Loeb RG: Monitor surveillance and vigilance of anesthesia residents. Anesthesiology 80: 527–533, 1994.
23. Loeb RG: Manual record keeping is not necessary for anesthesia vigilance. J Clin Monitoring 11: 9–13, 1995.
24. Chopra V, Gesink BJ, De Jong J, Bovill JG, Spierdijk J, Brand R: Does training on an anaesthesia simulator lead to improvement in performance? British Journal of Anaesthesia 73: 293–297, 1994.
25. Kanki B. G., Foushee H. C.: Communication as group process mediator of aircrew performance. Aviat Space Environ Med 60: 402–10, 1989.
26. Kanki B. G., Lozito S., Foushee H. C.: Communication indices of crew coordination. Aviat Space Environ Med 60: 56–60, 1989.
27. Orasanu J: Shared mental models and crew decision making, 46. Princeton University Cognitive Science Laboratory, 1990.
28. Foushee HC, Helmreich RL: Group interaction and flight crew performance, Human factors in aviation. Edited by Wiener EL, Nagel DC. San Diego, Academic Press, 1988, pp 189–228 .
29. Helmreich RL, Wilhelm JA, Gregorich SE, Chidester TR: Preliminary results from the evaluation of cockpit resource management training: performance ratings of flight crews. Aviat Space Environ Med 61: 576–579, 1990.
30. Helmreich RL, Wilhelm JA, Kello JE, Taggart WR, Butler RE: Reinforcing and evaluating crew resource management: evaluator/LOS instructor reference manual, Technical Manual 90–2, Revision 1. NASA/University of Texas, 1991.
31. Helmreich RL, Schaefer HG: Team performance in the operating room, Human Error in Medicine. Edited by Bogner MS. Hillsdale, NJ, Lawrence Erlbaum Associates, 1994, pp 225–253.
32. Gaba DM, Botney R, Howard SK, Fish KJ, Flanagn: Interrater reliability of performance assessment tools for the management of simulated anesthetic crises (abstract). Anesthesiology 81: A1277, 1994.

APPENDIX: NOTES ON THE UTILITY OF VIDEOTAPING IN HUMAN PERFORMANCE RESEARCH

Although it has drawbacks, videotape is an incredibly powerful tool for conducting human performance research.

- Videotapes constitute a *relatively* complete archival record of what was done, what was said, and what was happening
- The investigator can make multiple passes over the same tape, looking at different aspects of the same event(s)
- A re-analysis of the same events is possible by the original investigator or by other investigators to test new or "contradictory" hypotheses

The major disadvantage of videotape is the profound effort it takes to analyze the tapes. It typically takes 2–5 times as long as its original elapsed time to analyze a tape.

Here are a few tips for the best use of videotape:

- Obtain good quality AUDIO. A substantial fraction of data is in the audio not the video. Use professional-grade wireless microphone systems (not consumer grade) which are available at reasonable prices ($400 -$1400 per channel).
- Consumer-grade VIDEO (VHS, 8mm, SVHS, Hi8) is probably acceptable. The next step up (Betacam) is VERY expensive
- For multiple video views there are several choices:
  - Provide a separate VCR for each camera view
  - Use a video mixer (such as Videonics MX1) to insert one view "on top of" another (picture in picture)

PERFORMANCE ENHANCEMENT IN ANESTHESIA USING THE TRAINING SIMULATOR SOPHUS (PEANUTS)

John Jacobsen,[1] Per F. Jensen,[1] Doris Ostergaard,[2] Astrid Lindekær,[3] Anne Lippert,[3] and Peter Schultz[2]

[1]Department of Anesthesiology, Herlev Hospital
[2]Department of Anesthesiology, Gentofte Hospital
[3]Department of Anesthesiology, Glostrup Hospital
University of Copenhagen
Copenhagen County, Denmark

Although anesthesia today is a safe procedure, complications do arise. Several studies have tried to evaluate mortality and the frequency of complications in relation to operation and anesthesia.[1,2] In 14% of reported incidences the anesthesia in itself is considered to be a contributory factor. The major part of this factor is human error. Systematic collection of critical incidents "The Critical Incident Technique" was adopted from aviation and used for the first time in anesthesia by Cooper et al in 1978.[3] It was found like in aviation, that at least half of the reported critical incidents in the study was caused by human factors, mostly lack of knowledge about equipment in use and communication and/or leadership errors. In aviation this has lead to the development of simulators where it is possible to train both manual skills and aspects of communication, cooperation and leadership (the CRM concept). As there are some similarities between aviation and anesthesia the CRM concept has been transferred to anesthesia by Howard and Gaba by the use of simulators.[4] It has been shown that using simulators can improve performance.[5]

At Herlev hospital in Denmark the anesthesia simulator Sophus has been developed. A group of people interested in CRM has been established. Several courses have been conducted in the last three years implementing the above mentioned CRM concept in the Danish anesthesia community and there has been a great interest in this work. The Sophus group saw the possibility to address some of the problems in traditional theoretical improvement of medical education using the anesthesia simulator.

A project was designed for the residents in Copenhagen County with the objective to give theoretical education in the treatment of critical incidents and CRM principles followed by training in the anesthesia simulator. The working hypothesis was that the use of

Simulators in Anesthesiology Education, edited by Henson and Lee.
Plenum Press, New York, 1998.

103

the simulator would strengthen the implementation of the theoretical knowledge and improve the behavior of the anesthetist.

MATERIALS AND METHODS

The Subjects

Twenty-two residents working at the three major County university hospitals in Copenhagen participated after informed consent. In Denmark the education is divided in phases. The first phase consist of one year of formal anesthesia training as a junior resident. The second phase consist of two years of training as resident at a university hospital with formalized and specialized training in anesthesia, e.g. training in thoracic anesthesia, neuro-anesthesia. The third phase consist of 1½ year of training as senior resident with responsibilities as a leader of smaller anesthesia sections under supervision of a consultant.

The Simulator

The full-scale anesthesia simulator Sophus was set up in an operation theater with a simulator team acting as surgeons and nurses. The residents performance during the critical incidents was videotaped and these tapes were evaluated according to certain predefined criteria.

The Study Design

The study was randomized, single blinded with the residents in two groups. 12 residents (group B) received a full training program while 10 residents (group A) acted as a control group and received only the theoretical part of the program and a simulator demonstration session. All participants received instructions (algorithms) in diagnostic strategies and treatment of selected critical incidents. Furthermore they were educated in the importance of good coordination, leadership and communication during critical incidents. The study group participated in 6 simulator training sessions followed by debriefing sessions using videotapes of the simulator performance. The control group had a demonstration scenario to be familiarized with the setup. The following day all residents participated in a test scenario (abdominal aorta aneurysm). The flow diagram of the study is shown in Fig. 1. The scenario was videotaped and the tape evaluated by 3 specialists in anesthesia, who were unfamiliar to the grouping. The residents performance were characterized on a 4 point scale, where 1 is poor and 4 is best (Helmreich RL, personal communication). The groups were compared using a chi^2-test.

The control group was given the opportunity to train in the simulator after 3 months (and after the residents had performed in the second test).

RESULTS

There were no differences in different single parameters as establishment of team spirit, communication, coordination and leadership, situational awareness, decision making, consultation, instruction, special situations or overall impression of clinical anesthe-

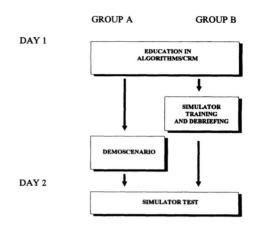

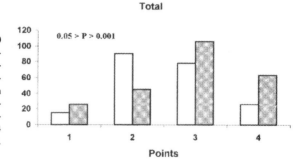

Figure 1. The flow of the participants in the study is shown. Group A is the control group and group B the study group. As a benefit the control group was given the opportunity to train similarly as the study group in the simulator after 3 months.

Figure 2. Total number of scores for all 10 parameters (team spirit, communication, coordination and leadership, situational awareness, decision making, consultation, instruction, special situations and overall impression of clinical anesthesia) in both groups (22 residents evaluated by 3 specialists). The residents performance were characterized on a 4 point scale, where 1 is poor and 4 is best. Shaded bars represents the study group.

sia, but when all parameters were considered together, group B performed better ($0.05 > P > 0.001$) (Fig. 2). In all parameters there was a tendency towards that the test group performed better than the control group. There were two "bad performers" both located in the test group.

DISCUSSION

We found that the effect of the theoretical education combined with the simulator training gave a better performance in the study group compared with the control group of residents. The two "bad performers" were both located in the test group which probably together with the relative small number of participants in the study we interpret is the reason for the lacking statistical difference in the single parameters. The subjective impression in the evaluator group was a clearly positive effect of the combination of the given theoretical education and the simulator training as also seen in the tendency to better performance in the single parameters. We have also considered that another problem is the difficulties of transformation of qualitative data into quantitative data.

REFERENCES

1. Petersen T, Eliasen K, Henriksen E. A prospective study of risk factors and cardiopulmonary complications associated with anaesthesia and surgery: risk indicators of cardiopulmonary morbidity. Acta Anaesthesiol Scand 1990; 34:144–55.
2. Duncan PG, Cohen MM, Tweed WA, Biehl D, Pope WD, Merchant RN, DeBoer D. The Canadian four centre study of anaesthetic outcome: III. Are anaesthetic complications predictable in day surgical practice? Can J Anaesth 1992; 39:440–5.
3. Cooper JB, Newbower RS, Long CD, McPeek B. Preventable anesthesia mishaps: a study of human factors. Anesthesiology 1978; 49:399–406.
4. Howard SK, Gaba DM, Fish KJ, Yang G, Sarnquist FH. Anesthesia crisis resource management training: teaching anesthesiologists to handle critical incidents. Aviation Space & Environmental Medicine 1992; 63:763–770.
5. Chopra V, Gesink BJ, De Jong J, Bovill JG, Spierdijk J, Brand R. Does training on an anaesthesia simulator lead to improvement in performance? Br J Anaesth 1994; 73:293–97.

14

JUMPSEATING[*] IN THE OPERATING ROOM

B. Sexton, S. Marsch, R. Helmreich, D. Betzendoerfer, T. Kocher,
D. Scheidegger, and the TOMS team

Departments of Anesthesia and Surgery
University of Basel
Basel, Switzerland

Department of Psychology
University of Texas at Austin
Austin, Texas, USA

INTRODUCTION

In safety sensitive cultures such as medicine, and especially in OR teams, communicating is critical. Williamson et al.'s report of 2000 critical incidents shows that 70% to 80% of medical mishaps are caused by human factors issues related to interpersonal interaction [1]. Data such as these represents what occurs in critical incidents, but does not provide us with insight as to communication in daily routine. Accordingly, the aim of this study was to assess the quality of communication between surgical and anesthesia teams in a teaching hospital.

METHODS

Trained and calibrated observers performed systematic observation of randomly selected surgical procedures from patient arrival until transfer to recovery room. Communication between anesthesia and surgical teams was observed. A four point interval scale classifies communication as being unacceptable or absent (1), barely acceptable/below expectations (2), meets expectations (3), outstanding (4). Absent communication refers to lack of both verbal and nonverbal communication (1). Communication representative of a 2 would be where the surgeon says "cutting" before he begins, but the communication is neither heard nor acknowledged by the Anesthesia team. An example of 3 would be when the surgeon asks "May we begin?" and becomes a definite answer. Ratings of 4 were given in instances where communication was maintained throughout the entire operation,

---

[*] "Jumpseating" is the technical term used to describe observations conducted in the cockpits of commercial and military aircraft. It stems from the cockpit "Jump Seat," or fold down seat located directly behind the pilot.

Simulators in Anesthesiology Education, edited by Henson and Lee.
Plenum Press, New York, 1998.

utilizing high levels of situational awareness, and initiative in communicating. Specific events were also noted.

RESULTS

90 operations were observed. In 20.3%, the communication was rated as either not present or unacceptable. More than fifty percent of the not present/unacceptable rating (1) was due to a failed communication of skin incision. Further, instances of the "1" rating stemmed from: failure to communicate removal of the aortic cross-clamp, implementation of Trendelenburg position without notifying the surgeon, complete lack of communication between the surgical and anesthesia teams, and failure to communicate insufficient regional anesthesia prior to incision. Communication was classified as 2, 3, and 4 in 53.2%, 24.1%, and 2.5% of the observations respectively.

DISCUSSION

Communication at the interface between anesthesia and surgical teams was classified as unacceptable/absent in approximately 20% of the observations. Moreover, in over 70% of the observed operations, the quality of communication was found to lie within the lower half of the scale. At present, the significance of these findings is uncertain. However, similar research in aviation has shown that superior performing teams communicate more and better than less effective teams [2].

REFERENCES

1. Williamson JA, Webb RK, Sellen A, Runciman WB, van der Walt JH. Human failure: an analysis of 2000 incident reports. Anaesth Intensive Care 1993;21:678–683.
2. Helmreich RL, Chidester TR, Foushee HC, Gregorich SA, Wilhelm JA. (1989b). How effective is cockpit resource management training? Issues in evaluating the impact of programs to enhance crew coordination. (NASA/Univ. of Texas Technical Report No. 89–2). Austin.

15

PARTICIPANT EVALUATION OF TEAM ORIENTED MEDICAL SIMULATION

B. Sexton, S. Marsch, R. Helmreich, D. Betzendoerfer, T. Kocher,
D. Scheidegger, and the TOMS team

Departments of Anesthesia and Surgery
University of Basel
Basel, Switzerland

Department of Psychology
University of Texas at Austin
Austin, Texas, USA

INTRODUCTION

The first high fidelity full scale operating room (OR) simulator has been installed at the University Hospital in Basel, Switzerland, and Team Oriented Medical Simulations (TOMS) have been conducted since December 1994. Simulation includes the complete OR team, comprising of surgical consultant, surgical resident, scrub nurse, anesthesia consultant, anesthesia resident, anesthesia nurse, and orderly, performing laparoscopic surgery on a mannequin undergoing general anesthesia. The aim of this study was to assess the participants' evaluation of their simulation session, and to determine whether the subgroups differed in their evaluation of the training.

METHODS

A simulation session consists of three phases, briefing, simulation, and debriefing. The briefing phase is essentially classroom training which presents the background and basic concepts to the participants, focusing on team coordination, communication and interface issues. This is then translated into specific behaviors during the simulation phase, where participants are given the opportunity to practice the concepts of team communication in both routine and critical simulated situations. These behaviors are then reinforced in the interactive debriefing using high quality video recordings of the simulation. At the end of a simulation session, each participant is asked to fill out a confidential post simulation evaluation questionnaire using a 10 point interval scale (1 = not at all valuable/realistic, 10 = extremely valuable/realistic).

Simulators in Anesthesiology Education, edited by Henson and Lee.
Plenum Press, New York, 1998.

RESULTS

128 questionnaires from participants of 22 full team simulations were analyzed. One-way analysis of variance was used to test for subgroup differences, the subgroups being, anesthesia consultants, anesthesia residents, anesthetic nurses, surgical consultants, surgical residents, surgical nurses, and orderlies. As there were no significant differences on any scale between the subgroups ($p > 0.2$ for all items), means and summary statistics are collapsed across all subgroups and sessions:

Nature of the evaluation item	Mean	SD	Median	Mode	Range
Realism of the scenario	7.06	1.27	7	8	3–10
Realism of team behavior	7.69	1.47	7.5	8	2–10
Value of briefing	8.39	1.91	9	10	3–10
Value of debriefing	9.07	1.11	10	10	5–10

DISCUSSION

The mean ratings for briefings and debriefings indicate very strong acceptance of the training. In fact, 89.4% of the 128 participants rated the value of the debriefing as 8, 9, or 10, reflecting a high level of the perceived importance of communication and interface issues in the OR. Realism of the scenario and team behavior also achieved favorable means, indicating that participants found not only their own behavior, but also the behaviors of others to highly resemble that of a real operating room. None of the subgroups differed in any of their ratings, suggesting that all groups benefited equally from the training. The results indicate that TOMS achieves a high level of realism for each of the constituents involved in OR patient management.

16

EVALUATION OF SIMULATOR USE FOR ANESTHESIA RESIDENT ORIENTATION

D. M. Barron and R. K. Russell

Department of Anesthesia
Brigham and Women's Hospital
Harvard Medical School
Boston, Massachusetts

Anesthesia simulators are perceived as important and desirable to first year anesthesia residents according to our study. Operating room simulators are being used in anesthesia training ranging from medical student clerkship to team performance training. Learning of basic anesthesia skills by first-year residents has been shown to be accelerated by simulator training.[1] We sought to evaluate residents' attitudes toward the use of a simulator during anesthesia residency orientation. Our evaluation was divided into four areas of interest, with the first concentration evaluating the use of a simulated operating room environment during orientation training. Specifically, did the simulator experience help in orientation to anesthesia residency both initially and when it was viewed after a significant period? Secondly, what is the learning preference of residents today? With the availability of numerous new teaching media (e.g., CD ROM, videotapes, computer simulation programs, simulators), do we need to incorporate these into our residency programs? Furthermore, do residents want these modalities available to them? And if so, do these supplant traditional lectures and workshops or are they are a supplement to textbook reading? Thirdly, after having the initial orientation at a simulator do residents desire more of this training and if so, would there be a willingness to sacrifice personal free time? Finally, does the presence of a simulator at a residency program in any way influence choice of a residency?

In July 1995, twelve first-year anesthesia residents from Brigham and Women's Hospital were randomly selected to attend a four-hour session at the Boston Anesthesia Simulation Center (BASC) in lieu of instruction in an operating room. All training sessions occurred during the first ten days of anesthesia residency. None of the residents had any significant prior training in anesthesia which was defined as more than a one month clerkship. The session consisted of a short review of the anesthesia machine, monitors, and preoperative assessment of the patient. Following this review, the residents were familiarized with the simulator environment. The residents were then allowed hands on management of three specific intraoperative physiological disturbances: hypoxemia, hypotension, and bradycardia. Cases were intermittently paused at key points intraoperatively

Simulators in Anesthesiology Education, edited by Henson and Lee.
Plenum Press, New York, 1998.

to allow for discussion of management. A self-report evaluation was performed following this initial session and again at eight months post experience.

The initial evaluation, performed immediately following the session, posted ratings which averaged 4.3/5 and 5/5 (1 = not very helpful to 5 = very helpful) for the review session and operating room simulation, respectively. Eleven of the twelve (91%) residents stated that the lecture was a good overview while one resident felt it was repetitive reflected material which had been addressed in orientation lectures. With respect to the operating room simulation, all twelve residents wished for more training including three (25%) who suggested that this session should be given to all residents during orientation. Similar positive results were gathered at the eight-month follow-up evaluation: all residents felt that simulation orientation training was valuable (12/12), enjoyable (11/11), had improved their confidence in starting their clinical training (12/12), and should be included as a planned component of anesthesia orientation (12/12). Eleven residents (91%) desired simulator training in addition to orientation lectures; only one resident desired simulator instruction instead of lecture.

With respect to learning modality preferences, six residents (50%) preferred new technologies, defined as simulators and CD ROM, compared to conventional technology, defined as lectures and workshops. Four residents (33%) felt equal affinity for both new and conventional teaching media and two residents (17%) preferred conventional methods. Simulator instruction was strongly preferred as a teaching modality when compared specifically to either workshop (10/12), lecture instruction (10/12), but only slightly preferred to textbook reading (6/11). Eleven residents (91%) indicated there were aspects of anesthesia training which could be taught better in a simulated environment compared to operating room case education

All the residents requested both future anesthesia training and the ability to reconstruct actual cases and review their management at the simulator. To accomplish these goals, 63% (7/11) responded that they were willing to attend the simulator after a night-call, and 75% (9/12) were willing to attend on their free time during a weekend.

With the decreasing number of anesthesia residency applicants, innovative and unique aspects which improve recruitment are worth pursuing. All of the residents felt that prospective applicants should be informed about the presence of a simulator at an anesthesia residency. Ninety-one percent (11/12) felt the presence of a simulator would enhance the appeal of a residency program.

Use of an anesthesia simulator as a teaching tool is an expense to anesthesia departments, both in terms of staff time and facility maintenance. A new teaching modality which offers a unique and enjoyable learning opportunity will likely enhance the educational experience and justify its own expense. Though self-reporting has many limitations (e.g., self-deception and responder bias), it is a qualitative measure of the attitude toward simulation training. Overall, the residents showed a very favorable reaction to both orientation and future anesthesia training at a simulator. The orientation training should be incorporated into anesthesia residency orientation, in addition to introductory lectures. The training during orientation was found to be valuable, enjoyable, and had improved residents' confidence in starting their clinical training in anesthesia. Interestingly, even the residents who stated that they did not enjoy training with new technologies compared to conventional technology did enjoy training in the simulator for orientation and wanted future training sessions. Perhaps familiarity with the new technologies makes them more appealing. Indeed, a point of interest, is the fact that the majority of the residents were willing to volunteer their personal time to obtain additional training at the simulator thus signifying its perceived importance in their training. Finally, the ability to train at a simulator was considered a desirable aspect of an anesthesia residency program. Since an important aspect of postgraduate training is the enthusiasm with which residents themselves pursue their education, anesthesia simulators can be a valuable tool in both anesthesiology resident recruitment and education.

REFERENCES

1. Good ML, Gravenstein JS, Mahla ME, White SE, Banner MJ, Carovano RG, Lemptang S. Can simulation accelerate the learning of basic anesthesia skills by beginning anesthesia residents? Anesthesiology 77(3A):A1133, Sept 1992.

17

INCORPORATION OF A REALISTIC ANESTHESIA SIMULATOR INTO AN ANESTHESIA CLERKSHIP

M. Pamela Fish[1,2] and Brendan Flanagan[1,2]

[1]Department of Anesthesia
Veterans Affairs Palo Alto Health Care System
Palo Alto, California
[2]Stanford University Medical Center
Stanford, California

1. INTRODUCTION

Following the opening of a dedicated anesthesia simulation center at the Veterans Affairs Palo Alto Health Care System in July 1995, we incorporated this realistic patient simulator into the current Stanford medical student clerkship in anesthesia. We report here our experiences with this course and on the response of our students to a simulation-based anesthesia education.

2. METHODS

The anesthesia clerkship at Stanford University Medical School is offered as a two week elective. Approximately 50 Stanford students and another 5–10 visiting students from other centers take this clerkship annually. Commencing October 1995, students taking the clerkship attended two half day sessions at the simulation center.

The first session was held on the first or second day of the clerkship. During this first session the students were oriented to the patient mannekin, patient monitors, emergency equipment, anesthesia machine and supply cart. Following this orientation the students then participated in several demonstrations. During these demonstrations they were responsible for the charting of vital signs from the monitors.

Session One

1. Orientation to simulator environment
2. Demonstrations:
   Apnea

Simulators in Anesthesiology Education, edited by Henson and Lee.
Plenum Press, New York, 1998.

Hypovolemia
Individual drugs
3. Induction of anesthesia

In the first demonstration the students rendered the mannekin apneic by the administration of thiopental and succinylcholine, initially without and then with pre-oxygenation. A graphic demonstration of the importance of pre-oxygenation resulted. The simulator also allowed the demonstration of the audible monitor alarms associated with hypoxia and apnea. The importance of an adequate circulating blood volume prior to inducing anesthesia was the aim of the second demonstration. The mannekin was subjected to a 600 ml blood loss over three minutes, during which one student pre-oxygenated the mannekin. Anesthesia was again induced using thiopental and succinylcholine, charting of vital signs by the students reinforcing the marked hypotension observed.

To improve their understanding of the properties of anesthetic drugs, the final demonstration consisted of performing a laryngoscopy to provide a 'noxious' stimulus to the mannekin. The resultant changes in vital signs were charted by the students. Thiopental, propofol, midazolam, fentanyl and succinylcholine were then administered individually. Following each administration of an individual drug the students again performed laryngoscopy as the stimulus, and the vital signs were recorded. This helped them to understand the effects these drugs were having on the hemodynamics of actual patients. The first session concluded with the students selecting and administering an anesthetic of their choice using the above agents. Their goal was to anesthetize the mannekin, perform laryngoscopy and intubate the trachea while keeping the mannekin hemodynamically stable.

Prior to attending the second session the students were given two case histories to evaluate. The first patient, a 19-year-old male, previously healthy, with a fractured femur

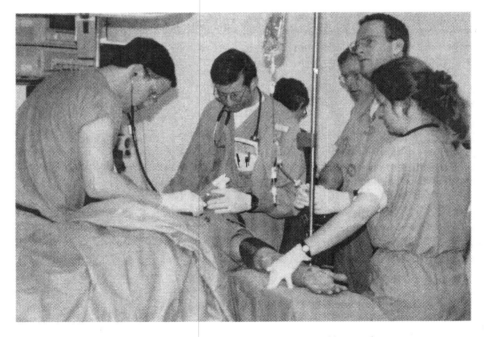

Figure 1. A typical group of medical students working together.

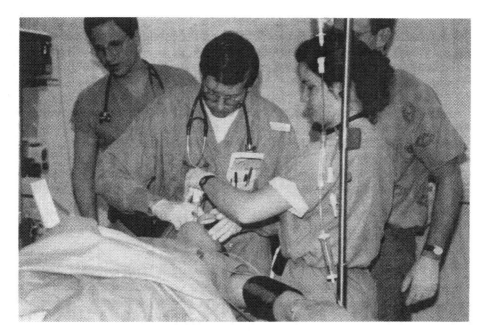

Figure 2. A successful induction!

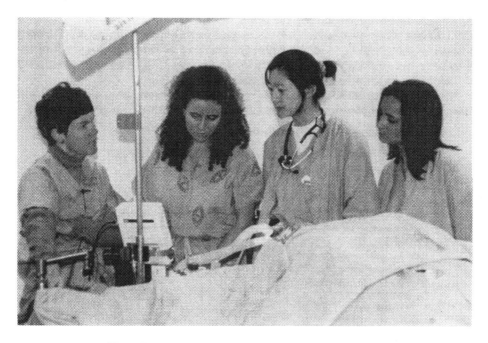

Figure 3. The students receive feedback on their performance.

following an MVA. The second patient, a 75-year-old male with hypertension and COPD, presenting for pinning of a fractured hip. This second session commenced with a discussion of potential anesthetic problems for these two patients and plans for their anesthetic management. The students worked through which drugs to use and their dosage. They allocated themselves specific roles, and then questioned and examined the "patient". Following a machine and equipment check, they placed their choice of patient monitors and commenced fluid replacement.

Following the induction phase, time was allowed for the students to become familiar with the case; a critical incident, such as atelectasis or myocardial ischemia, was then simulated. Working as a group, the students then formulated a diagnosis and instituted initial corrective therapy.

Following each scenario, feedback was given to the students on the positive aspects of their management, while any obvious problems or misconceptions were explained.

Session Two

1. Case discussion
2. Preparation and management of case
3. Review of management

Before and after each session, participating students completed anonymous questionnaires regarding the role of the anesthesia simulator in their medical student clerkship.

3. RESULTS

All students considered both Sessions One and Two to be educational. 31 students considered their time better spent in the simulator during Session One while Session Two had 30 students preferring the simulator over the operating room for time well spent. For both sessions the majority of students thought that they accomplished more than in the same time in the operating room., especially in Session Two. All students stated they would attend future sessions if they were made available.

The positive way these students viewed their simulator sessions is shown below. The students comments emphasize some of the advantages of simulation-based education.

Representative comments written by the students:

- "Session on first day is an effective introduction to anesthesia"
- "Clinical scenarios are an excellent way for me to learn"

Table 1. Evaluation by students of simulator sessions

Question	Yes	No	Undecided
Demonstrations educational?	32	0	0
Session suitable for level of training?	31	1	0
Time would be better spent in OR?			
Session One	0	31	1
Session Two	1	30	1
Accomplished more than same time in OR?			
Session One	22	8	2
Session Two	27	3	2
Would come to future sessions	32	0	0

- "More comfortable in real OR, because I can't screw up there!"
- "At the student level the simulator offers some hands on experience vs. the OR"
- "Being in charge rather than watch residents was very helpful in learning"
- "I think session two complements the OR experience effectively"
- "I think all aspects of session were instructive—it felt very real!"

4. DISCUSSION

We developed simulator-based teaching sessions as an adjunct to the clerkship in anesthesia. The students attending these sessions were unanimous in their opinion that the anesthesia simulator added a new and complementary dimension to the anesthesia clerkship. The opportunity to take responsibilty for all aspects of the anesthetic plan, including problem management, was a unique aspect of the simulator session. Working in groups, the students responded well to the critical events presented. The real-time dynamic situations created allowing them a better feeling for the nuances of anesthesia. Our course continues to evolve as we gain experience and feedback. The positive response received to date from the students suggests it will continue as an important part of the anesthesia clerkship at our institution.

18

COMPUTER ANALYSIS OF CEREBROVASCULAR HEMODYNAMICS DURING INDUCTION OF ANESTHESIA

A. Bekker,[1] S. Wolk,[2] H. Turndorf,[1] and A. Ritter[2]

[1]New York University Medical Center
Department of Anesthesiology
New York, New York
[2]New Jersey Institute of Technology
Newark, New Jersey

OBJECTIVE

The purpose of this project was to develop a computer model of cerebrovascular hemodynamics interacting with a pharmacokinetic drug model to examine the effects of various stimuli during anesthesia on cerebral blood flow and intracranial pressure.

METHODS

The mathematical model of intracranial hemodynamics is a seven compartment constant volume system [1]. A series of resistances relate blood and cerebrospinal fluid fluxes to pressure gradients between compartments. Arterial, venous, and tissue compliances are also included. Autoregulation is modeled by transmural pressure dependent arterial-arteriolar resistance. The effect of a drug (thiopental) on cerebrovascular circulation was simulated by a variable arteriolar-capillary resistance. Thiopental concentration, in turn, was predicted by a three-compartment pharmacokinetic model. The effect site compartment was introduced to account for disequilibrium between thiopental plasma and biophase concentration [2]. The simulation program is written in VisSim[R] dynamic simulation language for an IBM-compatible PC. The model was validated by comparing simulation results with available experimental observations.

RESULTS

Series of computer simulations of the typical induction process for a simulated patient with normal and increased ICP were performed. Administration of the induction dose

Simulators in Anesthesiology Education, edited by Henson and Lee.
Plenum Press, New York, 1998.

121

of thiopental (5 mg/kg) resulted in reduction of ICP up to 20%. However, rapid redistribution of thiopental and cerebral autoregulation limited the duration of this effect to less than three minutes. Subsequent laryngoscopy, which is associated with an increase in the mean arterial pressure (50 torr in our study), causes acute intracranial hypertension, exceeding the initial ICP. Computer simulation predicted that this untoward effect can be minimized by an additional dose of thiopental prior to intubation.

DISCUSSION

We have developed a mathematical model of cerebrovascular circulation, on which both prediction of hemodynamic responses and evaluation of drug effect can be made. The effects of various stimuli on CBF and ICP in a normal and a compromised (non-autoregulated) cerebral vasculature have been compared. It was concluded that the presented computer simulation permits comparison of drug administration schedules to control ICP and preserve CBF during various phases of anesthesia.

REFERENCES

1. Ursino M. Computer analysis of the main parameters extrapolated from the human intracranial basal artery blood flow. Comp Biomed Research 1990; 23: 542–561
2. Stanski D., Maitre P. Population pharmacokinetics and pharmacodynamics of thiopental: the effect of age revisited. Anesthesiology 1990; 72: 412–421

INDEX

ACCESS: *see* Simulators, full-scale
ACLS: *see* Advanced cardiac life support
ACRM: *see* Anesthesia crisis resource management
Advanced cardiac life support, 15, 16, 63
Aircraft simulation: *see* Aviation
Airway management, 4, 10, 25, 27, 30–32, 63, 82, 116
Anaphylaxis, 63, 64
Anesthesia care team, 29, 31, 33
Anesthesia crisis resource management, 4, 23, 26, 42, 44
Anesthesia machine, 4, 25, 31, 39, 41
ASC: *see* Simulators, screen-only
Attention: *see* Vigilance
Aviation, 1–3, 40, 45–46, 94, 99

Behavior: *see* Team performance
BODY simulation: *see* Simulators, screen-only

CASE: *see* Simulators, full-scale
Certification, 30, 46, 86
Clerkships: *see* Curriculum, medical students
Clinical education, 15–16, 23, 27, 29–30, 32–26, 67, 94–95, 99, 101; *see also* Curriculum
CME: *see* Continuing medical education
Cockpit resource management (CRM), 2–3; *see also* Aviation
Cognitive knowledge, 4, 33, 35, 60, 62, 95
Communication, 2, 3, 5, 51, 55, 76, 101, 103, 107
Competence: *see* Certification
Computer
    hardware, 10, 23, 42, 75–76, 91–92
    personal, 6, 43, 44, 75–76
    programming, 66, 67, 70
    software, 75–84, 89–91, 121, 122
    skills, 75, 89
Continuing medical education, 43, 87
Costs, simulator programs, 85, 89, 91–92
Crew resource management, 1, 3, 5, 44–45, 103
Critical care education, 15, 16, 41
Critical incident reporting system (CIRS), 6, 51
Critical incidents, 2, 40, 42, 44, 46, 51–52, 87, 93–95, 103, 118

Curriculum
    medical students, 11, 15–22, 23–28, 115–116, 118
    nurse anesthesia students, 29–37
    residents, 11, 23–28, 42, 45, 86, 104, 112

Debriefing, 6; *see also* Anesthesia crisis resource management, Team oriented medical simulation
Decision making, 1, 6, 31–33, 36, 59
Differential diagnosis, 24, 30, 34, 61, 63, 99, 118
Difficult airway algorithm: *see* Airway management
Drugs, 6, 63, 64, 66, 82, 118, 122

Education, 30, 33–34, 86, 105; *see also* Curriculum
Educational goals, 9, 58, 66
Emergency medicine, 42, 90
Ergonomics, 40, 47
Errors, 35, 52, 99; *see also* Human factors
Evaluation
    equipment, 43
    performance, 9, 40, 43, 59, 86–87
    teaching, 34–35

Faculty, 16, 33, 36, 57, 65, 67, 70, 82, 88–89, 90, 92
Fidelity of simulators, 20, 52, 95; *see also* Realistic simulation
Flight crews: *see* Aviation
Full-scale simulators: *see* Simulators, full-scale
Funding of simulator programs, 44, 85, 87–91

Gas Man: *see* Simulators, screen-based

Hardware: *see* Computer
Heart sounds, 75
Hemodynamic variables, 12, 43, 52, 81–82, 116, 121–122
Human errors: *see* Errors
Human factors, 2, 3, 4, 5, 51, 96, 98, 103, 107
Human Patient Simulator (HPS), 15, 16, 17–21, 42, 63, 64, 76–78; *see also* Simulators, full-scale
Human performance, 93–101
Hyperthermia: *see* Malignant hyperthermia
Hypervigilance, 95

Instructors: *see* Faculty
Intensive care, 47
Interface, human-machine, 40, 44, 45
Intubate: *see* Airway management

Laryngospasm: *see* Airway management
Learning objectives, 58–59, 60–63, 72
Legal aspects, 90, 91
Line oriented flight training (LOFT), 2, 4
Leiden anesthesia simulator (LAS): *see* Simulators, full-scale
Loral Corporation: *see* Simulators, full-scale

Malignant hyperthermia, 45, 78
Manikin: *see* Mannequin
Mannequin, 6, 10, 16, 20, 41–43, 45, 47, 53, 54, 95
Mathematical models, 12, 27, 65, 68, 72, 75–84, 95, 121
Medical Education Technologies (METI): *see* Human Patient Simulator and simulators, full-scale
Medical students: *see* Curriculum
Mental workload, 96–98
Models, 6, 31, 66–68, 73, 78, 82
Monitors
   capnogram, 12
   EKG, 12, 63, 75, 97
   PA catheter, 81
   pulse oximeter, 43
Morbidity and mortality: *see* Quality assurance
Motor skills, 32, 44, 75, 103

Nurse anesthetists, 29, 30, 36

Objective structured clinical examination (OSCE), 20–21
Observation, 40, 55, 94, 107
Operating room, 3, 5–6, 15–16, 32–33, 40, 43, 51–52, 86, 88, 109

Patient, (real or simulated), 6, 32–33, 36, 40, 47, 52, 54, 66–67, 77–78, 93–94
Pat Sim simulator: *see* Simulators, full-scale
Performance measurement, 3, 86, 95, 97–101, 105

Physiology, 11–12, 14, 16, 65, 70, 85, 95
Pilots: *see* Aviation
Pre-programmed scenarios, 65–66, 68, 76, 82
Problem based learning (PBL), 11, 58, 59

Quality assurance, 36, 39, 45

Realistic simulation, 20, 93–101, 115–116
Real time, 77, 119
Regional anesthesia, 29
Research with simulators, 31, 87, 90, 95–96
Residents: *see* Curriculum
Resources: *see* Funding

Scenarios, designing, 11–12, 58–59, 78–84
Shock, 75
Simulated patients, examples, 12–14, 63, 78, 81–82
Simulator facilities, 3, 6, 24, 32, 35–36, 44, 46, 65, 85, 88, 91
Simulators
   full-scale, 6, 42–44, 65, 76–78, 103–106
   screen-only, 34, 41–42
   virtual reality, 45–46
Situational awareness, 1, 6, 35, 36
Skills, 16, 18, 21, 30, 35, 40, 51–52, 86, 99
Sophus anesthesia simulator: *see* Simulators, full-scale
Software: *see* Computers
Surgery, 4–6, 44–45, 51

Task analysis, 97–98
Team oriented medical simulation (TOMS), 44, 46, 51–55, 110
Team performance, 2, 3, 6, 54, 55, 99, 104, 109
Technological aspects, 40, 52, 76–78, 87, 112

Videotaping, 6, 55, 102, 109
Vigilance, 95, 96–98
Virtual Anesthesiology Training Simulator System (VATSS), 42, 76–78; *see also* Simulators, full-scale
Virtual reality, 44–45, 47

Wilhelm Tell simulator: *see* Simulators, full-scale

Breinigsville, PA USA
04 October 2010
246694BV00009B/2/A